Social Aspects of HIV

Series Editors
Peter Aggleton
Seth Kalichman
Susan Kippax
Richard G. Parker
John de Wit

Since the start of the epidemic, HIV and AIDS have fired the imaginations of social as well as medical and public health scientists. This innovative series of books offers a setting in which to publish the very best of social scientific thinking and research. The Social Aspects of HIV series of books offers readers authoritative introductions and overviews, together with summaries of enduring and cutting edge concerns. The series is international and multidisciplinary in focus, including contributions from psychology, sociology, anthropology, education, economic, political and social theory, and international development. Individual volumes offer scholarly overviews of key topics and concerns but also address 'big issues' relevant to HIV prevention, treatment and care. Sexual and drug-related practices; adherence; disclosure; and stigma and discrimination are among topics focused upon, alongside broader cultural, political and social responses to the epidemic, including globalisation and internationalisation. The political economy of AIDS, links to broader questions of sexual health and rights, and the progressive biomedicalisation of the response, will also be among key issues examined.The series will appeal to those working in public health, health psychology, medical sociology, medical anthropology, health promotion, social work and international development. Individual volumes will be relevant to students, teachers, researchers and practitioners within each of these disciplines as well as program developers and managers working across a variety of contexts.

More information about this series at http://www.springer.com/series/11922

Hakan Seckinelgin

The Politics of Global AIDS

Institutionalization of Solidarity, Exclusion of Context

Springer

Hakan Seckinelgin
Department of Social Policy
London School of Economics
and Political
London, UK

ISSN 2509-6559 ISSN 2509-6567 (electronic)
Social Aspects of HIV
ISBN 978-3-319-46011-6 ISBN 978-3-319-46013-0 (eBook)
DOI 10.1007/978-3-319-46013-0

Library of Congress Control Number: 2016955093

Printed on acid-free paper

This Springer imprint is published by Springer Nature
The registered company is Springer International Publishing AG
The registered company address is: Gewerbestrasse 11, 6330 Cham, Switzerland

For my mother Beyhan and Damien

Preface

Field Notes from Global AIDS

On this particular day, we were visiting a prison outside of Bujumbura (Burundi). I had heard that a number of people had organized themselves as an HIV-positive support group to help each other in the prison, so I wanted to talk to them for my research. The meeting had been arranged through a local human rights lawyer who worked for a non-governmental organization (NGO) and was aware of the group.

We arrived at the prison. It was outside Bujumbura, but not too far away in the middle of the countryside. My first impression was that there were too many people and it was really crowded. We were taken through the corridors to see the prison administrator first, women and men were separated, but both sides of the prison were very noisy, and many people were behind bars; inside people were cooking, I could smell the fire and food, it was very busy, and the corridors were hard to pass through. The person who was facilitating this meeting – George (a pseudonym) – was telling us that the prison had at the time over three times the prisoners that it should have contained. We were taken into an area a bit like a shed with an open front looking to the front yard of the prison. Three prisoners were allowed to come and talk to us there: One of them was the young man who had initiated the support group for HIV-positive prisoners. He talked about how they started the group to help themselves because there were no other resources to support them in the prison. They were cooking food and selling it to make money to support their HIV-related needs. He said that they did not need to go out and look for people to join them because word of mouth brought people to their group. He added that 'many people don't know they have HIV and get really sick while in the prison, and they are diagnosed, but there are no real resources to support them after the diagnosis, and some don't get diagnosed at all, we just know the signs'. The main problem he said, pointing the oldest man in the group, was that, for instance, 'he is really sick; he needs to get proper treatment outside, but he cannot get out from the prison since for months he is waiting to see the judge', to be told whether there will be a case against him or not. 'There are so many people waiting to be charged for months; there are many people like this; some even die in the prison waiting to see the judge'. Given that 'many people don't come from this area, they don't have relatives to come and support them with food', so people were reliant on the very little that can get within the prison. That's 'why we started this group. But it is not enough. We were told that if you are sick like us, they will release us, but still nothing has happened'.

George also explained that sometimes the group got help from international NGOs but that this was not enough. I asked whether people acquired HIV in the prison. I had to ask this question very carefully. Given the gender segregation, it was a sensitive issue touching on same sex-related taboos. He said that they thought some women might catch HIV as there were ways of having sex with women even if they were living in separate parts of the prison. Then I asked how about the men. He was more cautious but said that 'younger men, who are not from this area, work for older and richer men. They cook for them, clean the place they sleep; they become dependent' on the relationship to survive, and 'sometimes they are very close' because otherwise they would have had nothing to survive. He stopped at that. It was a difficult set of interviews, and it was even harder to think what one could do to influence change in these circumstances and who I should talk to… (December 2008).

It was 2010 and I was in Vienna (Austria) for a meeting of the *Thinking Politically* group held at the XVIII International AIDS Conference. The meeting seemed to be a joint initiative between the International AIDS Society (IAS) and UNAIDS. Dennis Altman and Kent Buse were the planners and, I assumed, the main motivators behind the initiative. They were really enthusiastic and had gathered together a group of political scientists from across the globe. We had a good meeting, discussing different ways of motivating political science research on HIV and how to bring existing research in this area to engage with the epidemic. Our concern though was also with the broader context of the IAS and how best to bring relevant research to the attention of policymakers. It was a discussion about political science but also touched on the strategy of how to engage with various groups from this particular perspective. Dennis and Ken did a good job in arranging a 'networking' lunch, which included some important and influential policy actors. One of them, a person who was at the top of the policy chain, in a discussion turned around and said that the main problem with AIDS today was its over-medicalization. I could not believe my ears; I was rather perplexed thinking that medicalization did not happen naturally. I was wondering what was being done to address this issue given that the person was in position of responsibility. It was rather an odd way to start the conference process. I was buzzing with ideas from the meeting as we had had a good discussion, but I also did not know what to think about this statement concerning medicalization in relation to the conference programme… (July 2010).

After a few weeks in Gulu (Uganda), I managed to go to the hospital to look at their HIV clinic. The hospital there was very important as it not only provided health-related services to a wide area but also, as I was told by the priest who had taken me to the hospital, because a lot of people had sought refuge in the hospital during the Lord's Resistance Army (LRA) troubles. There were a lot of people waiting outside. He mentioned that some of these people came from South Sudan every morning as this was the biggest facility available. The inside was also busy, with many people who must have been relatives sleeping outside the wards. The HIV unit, around a courtyard garden, was quieter; it must have been the time of the day. I met the doctor responsible for the unit. He was very welcoming and talked about ARV provision and other issues they were facing. It seemed that they were able to engage their patients in a structured way to provide ARV, and he said that the hospital had good relationships with its patients. Then he began to talk about other problems: '[But] we sometimes received letters from people from villages – not near here in the bush – asking us to give them ARVs. They say that they were on treatment provided by an NGO, but for a few months now they have not had anyone coming from the NGO to give them treatment, so they don't have medicine and that they are worried'. The problem was that 'we have limited supplies related to the number of patients we have, [so] I cannot suddenly provide medicine to unexpected others'. This would have put "my patients'" treatment into danger'.

Another problem he highlighted was that since the peace, people were now travelling more so they could get access to treatment, and they often travel elsewhere in the country: 'We don't know what happens to these people, whether they then get access to treatment elsewhere or they stop'. He went on, 'We also have problems with men'; women get their treatment for a month, and then they came back earlier to get more. He said that 'men are using their wives' pills knowing that if she has AIDS, I must too, but they do not want to come to the hospital. This is also making the management of treatment difficult'. It struck me that these were all important challenges in this remote part of Uganda. Also I was not sure how things would work out in the future as the closure of The AIDS Support Organization (TASO) treatment centres was being discussed. He did not say a lot about the Sudanese patients, but I wondered whether they were also receiving treatment through this hospital, which was resourced through the Ugandan (Global Fund) mechanism… (August 2012).

Sitting through the panel presentations (at the 2012 AIDS Conference, Washington D.C., USA) was tedious. Speakers made massive generalizations from rather small sample groups to talk about the usefulness of what they were doing for most people who were at risk of HIV. This was worrisome. I just didn't see what would make their arguments work elsewhere. Presenters needed to argue why their claims were relevant. Major assumptions were being made about adherence and adherence over a lifetime. Speakers were also making jumps from scientific outcomes to policymaking and guidelines. I wondered if having the scientific results really justified peoples' competence to make policy. In this particular panel, discussion of the treatment cascade was interesting. But there was not much discussion to explain why at each point in the cascade a percentage of those on the cascade were lost and what was going on to cause this at each step. This was interesting to think about: If this described the situation in the USA with its massive resources, what might it suggest in much poorer countries? What would their cascade look like, and how would one explain the drop-off at each step? Interesting … I was not sure how at the same conference discussion of the goal of 15 million by 2015 under treatment could make sense taking into account the causes and implications of drop-off in the cascade as shown in another panel. Did these people talk to each other? … I had just seen Rachel (Deacon, my PhD student at the time) who also shared her frustration about the conference. She was surprised about the lack of social science input, but even more so by the lack of social science understanding. I had to say ‘welcome to the club!’ (July 2012).

In South Sudan, we were going to go back to the refugee camp in Ezo as we had agreed with the administrator there. They had recommended we also go and see a guy in the international NGO who was dealing with the health issues in the camp. That same morning, we were told by the person who brought us here that on the other side of the road was the Central African Republic, literally over the road from where we were then sitting. The Congo [DRC] was a bit further away, but it was also within walking distance, as the local market was on the border there. The camp itself was a bit further away from the square, perhaps a few miles away in the bush. It had a reception area and immediately I noticed that against the left-hand wall, there was a box, clearly for condoms. They said they put the supplies there and that anyone could come and pick them up when they wanted. I could not stop myself from opening the box to look inside; it was empty, and the administrator said with a little smile, ‘we are waiting for supplies’. The camp appeared to be managed by International SOS, an international NGO, on behalf of UNHCR … The day before, we had noticed that there were a lot of people around. On this day, we first interviewed the international NGO guy who dealt with the health in the camp. He was friendly. He said that often with patients, nutrition was a problem so that they provided it particularly to children. He said that as all refugees were registered they were able to keep track of them but that sometimes they would see new sick people in the camp and that these were not registered. It was clear from his remarks that there was a lot of health-/AIDS-related movement between Congo and the camp. He said that HIV numbers were generally high and that most people were tested ‘once they arrived in Ezo and realized this, but some also arrived knowing that they were HIV-positive had but never had any treatment in the Congolese side’ as resources in the conflict area were very limited. For tests and other clinical interventions, they needed to go to the hospital in Nzara (about 2–3 h drive from the camp depending on the road and weather conditions). He added that ‘every few months we do awareness activity and get them to test’. After this conversation, I thought what he said must be correct as in the camp it was easy to talk about HIV and AIDS; people were very open about their status and needs even when others were around. In conversation, a number of people said that ‘it started in Congo’ and that they learned they were ‘HIV-positive here’. Talking to a group of women in their mid-20s to early 30s, one of them said that ‘there are problems with [the] hospital and its distance from the camp’. She said that she went to the hospital but never got proper medicine for what she needed, just always the same pill for headaches. But then two others began to talk about the HIV medications and care they get in the camp and the fact that they talk about this to their husbands. This was fascinating, as the two clinics they were talking about were so different: The first person was talking about the original clinic in the camp dealing with health in general, but which had now been moved away from the camp, while the other women were talking about the HIV clinic to which they were taken regularly for their treatment needs. The difference between these clinics was something to think about… (December 2012).

I met the main fundraiser guy in Geneva (Switzerland) to discuss whether it would be possible to raise some funds to support some of the main social science-related activities we were planning for the Melbourne World AIDS Conference in 2014. He was very direct and said that the funding of the conference is generally difficult and also that they realized that people 'don't want to fund social sciences; they don't know what it means in relation to AIDS'… (November 2013).

After asking a few people, we managed to set up a meeting with a local HIV-positive people's community organization. I met with two reps in their office, a flat in a block of apartments not too far from the centre of Yangon (Myanmar). They talked a lot about access issues and the complications of having different organizations providing treatment and also about the existing unmet needs. They said that 'most of the time there is a service quality difference between International NGOs (INGOs), local NGOs and the national programme. The national programme provided only treatment; some national NGOs provide food package and counselling space'. What was interesting was that when talking about stigma, they made reference to issues such as 'the work place, in schools for children, for housewives and at the public hospitals'. After asking a few more questions about the groups that were most stigmatized, they talked about men who have sex with men (MSM). I got the impression that this was not an easy thing even for this group to talk about: 'MSM has high stigma. In hospitals they don't want to give MSM [a] proper examination. For MSM, it is also difficult to have access to ARVs. These are issues for medical staff. They give reasons like *they are MSM; IDUs are not stable people, so they cannot control themselves*. They don't want to deal with them [MSM and IDUs (Injection Drug Users)]. They are not ready to change their minds'. This was in line with what I heard later the same day from a doctor working in a medical INGO. He said access to MSM was 'very, very difficult – as access to them to conduct research was very mediated. MSM do not trust people to keep them anonymous'. I also had a discussion with an international AIDS expert who directly said that 'MSM is a problem. MSM is a problem because, normally, talking about sex is not accepted. Sex is an issue in a very conservative society. They just don't talk about it. They also consider MSM from the perspective of the receptive partner and also more in relation to transgender. Policy intake on this issue is very difficult; the research is difficult'. Interestingly on that same day, everyone talked about the difficulties of reaching groups, difficulties that were clearly based on existing norms and values. Compared to MSM, sex workers were more visible, but they also faced similar problems in relation to service access because people were not interested in their issues. One NGO leader said that she had taken some people from the parliament, lawyers, to Melbourne for the AIDS Conference for them to see how other countries worked with sex workers and that it was helpful in the end … but it was not very clear how all of these would relate to the imminent political change in the country. Would local sociocultural prejudices change if the regime changes? According to some, no not really (October 2014).

The return from every field visit is crowded with anxieties and questions about the issues observed. The difficulty is to see how some of these dynamics can change to allow people to live the lives they want to lead. This always requires one to think about what needs to happen in terms of the politics and policy within which AIDS is approached. However, I have also observed over the years a gap between diverse experiences of HIV and AIDS in the field and the discussions of HIV I have been involved in at the international level while participating in conferences or discussions with key policy actors. In these discussions, I have always thought that people are very dedicated and driven to tackle the disease wherever it occurs. At the same time, I have always thought that ordinary people live their lives and experience HIV in particular ways. These field observations have also taken place in what gradually has become an area of study, now commonly known as global health. In this field, HIV has become an archetypical global health issue. This created for me an analytic question: What is global about HIV in the lives of people I have observed in the field? It is true that their lives intersect with the more international dimensions of AIDS, but via a series of encounters that does not represent the entirety of the way people live as observed in my fieldwork. In poorer countries, people may experience the global aspects of AIDS through NGOs, clinics, the media and more gradually through schools. But these encounters do not represent the entirety of infected and affected persons' experiences with HIV. However, I have also come to realize that, for the international community of scholars and policymakers concerned with HIV, these encounters have come to construct who infected and affected people are and what their lives are about. Through an HIV and AIDS lens, different lives are thereby brought together as a community, a community of concern and for policy action.

Global AIDS as Field of Research Interest

The brief field notes above identify some of the different dynamics at work in diverse places, yet it is also possible to observe within them a common approach to dealing with AIDS overall. What I will call the Global AIDS system facilitates the focusing of research and public attention on particular parts of the world and particular topics. These then become different issues of concern for Global AIDS policy. Throughout this process, however, the Global AIDS approach itself escapes from being researched as a frame of reference or as an institutionalized process in which organizational actors develop policy priorities that affect people's lives deeply as part of their HIV-related experience. So, how best do we think about Global AIDS as a part of people's experience of HIV/AIDS? This question and the observations that led to it highlight a key issue, namely, how does the Global AIDS system differentiate the 'field' – into research and into HIV and the expertise that produces priorities, policies and plans for the future. By focusing closely on this differentiation, the field can become a context of discovery, a mini-laboratory if you like. In this book, I argue that this process of differentiation – between science and application – is a problem and that this latter setting should be opened up for research as a legitimate part of HIV- and AIDS-related analytical questioning.

Another issue that I have encountered concerns the analytic tools available for thinking and understanding research observations obtained from different sites: How best do I observe the specific and then derive their implications for policy thinking? The answers to these questions are nearly always those already provided by the Global AIDS system in the form of policy-relevant conceptual frameworks. This creates further questions: What are the ways in which the 'givenness' of this system frames the problem and people's lives? Are the given analytical orientations relevant, who are they relevant to, and do they allow people's experiences and voices to influence and change the policies that target them? So, the question for me is not only about the policy impact of the Global AIDS system in its organizational aspects but also about the way in which it conceptually frames thinking on AIDS in relation to real people's lives. In order to unpack these issues, this book focuses in on the knowledge production processes that are an essential part of the Global AIDS system.

The book's metatheoretical orientation is closely related to my earlier work (2006). In that work, I developed a specific analytic lens to think about HIV and AIDS, which moves us away from looking at the problems of HIV from the point of view of the international organizations that try to align people's responses to international AIDS policies. Instead, I argue that policy thinking should start from the way in which the disease is experienced by real people in different contexts of their lives. Karin Flikschuh (2014: 1), a political theorist, advocates for 'philosophical fieldwork as a possible corrective to our current state of ignorance regarding the thoughts and views of distant others in the context of global normative theorising'. Her writing is akin to my own thinking. For her, fieldwork is a conceptual engagement in relation to distant others. She writes:

> [By] 'distant others' I do not mean the 'global poor' but our academic peers who work within moral and political contexts distinct from ours and whom we tend not to consult in our global theorising: distant intellectually as much as geographically. (2014: 1)

This book is an attempt to provide a way of thinking about Global AIDS and its normative framework from the position of being an intellectual other than within the global system. This orientation arises, similar to Flikschuh, from a concern with the continued emergency-logic which aims to 'solve' the AIDS problem in a constant present that does not allow for theoretical enquiry about the nature of the Global AIDS itself and one which leads to the establishment of particular ways of doing AIDS as 'a value system' (2014: 2). The way in which this process is naturalized as an intervention in people's lives requires questioning.

In this book, then, by developing an analysis on the relationship between the institutionalization of particular policy processes and actors and the knowledge production process in general, I am interested in the implications of the Global AIDS lens as it seeks to make sense of different people's lives in different places. This requires us to consider the implications of this process for those living lives that intersect both with HIV and with this global system of policy, which I call Global

AIDS. This is a vast area for research, and no single book can provide a comprehensive or definitive answer to these questions. The aim here though is to think innovatively, outside the box, and to raise questions that provide new ways to do research on HIV and AIDS. The analysis is based on multiple sources of knowledge based on field experiences, participatory observations from within the global policy process on implementation issues, other forms of research and the existing literature. The Global AIDS system has major implications for how people living with HIV sustain their lives and achieve their aspirations. A driving question, however, is whether the Global AIDS system as it has emerged over time has the expertise and the capacity to maintain change in its engagement with different people across different places. As I will show, under the impact of need for sustainability, this is far from an abstract question.

London, UK Hakan Seckinelgin

Acknowledgements

It has taken several years of research in many different parts of the world to write this book. I am deeply grateful to those who discussed their lives and experiences with me along the way. I am indebted to a large number of people. Sharing their views and hopes in these discussions over the years, they have made me think about HIV, AIDS and everyday lives in different ways. This book could not have been without them. Similarly, I have been fortunate to be part of research and policy processes that have informed my thinking about HIV and its consequences. I thank each and every one of the many people who I have encountered in these processes. More specifically over the years, I have discussed with or have observed discussions among a number of colleagues. I learned much from these exchanges. I thank in particular Dennis Altman, Judy Auerbach, Tony Barnett, Kent Buse, Cathy Campbell, Flora Cornish, Catherine Hankins, Tim Hildebrandt, Armine Ishkanian, Jennifer Klot, Guillaume Lachenal, David Lewis, Dana Rosenfeld, Lisa Ann Richey, Justin Pankhurst, Ulla Pape, Bruno Spire and Per Strand. I also benefited from our discussions in the LSE Evidence Group. I thank Nancy Cartwright, Jeremy Hardie, Eleonora Montuschi and Eileen Munro. I also thank the series editors of *Social Aspects of HIV Series* by Springer Press Peter Aggleton, Seth Kalichman, Susan Kippax, Richard G. Parker and John de Wit for their interest in my work. I am particularly grateful to Peter Aggleton who as the series editor on this book provided insightful, critical and detailed comments. These made the book much better, working with him was a master class. I also thank Bernadette Deelen-Mans and Evelien Bakker at Springer for their support from the inception of this project. I started to write the book during sabbatical leave from my university, and I very much thank Françoise and William Fennell for allowing me so generously to stay at *rue de l'Alboni* as I finalized the draft during this time. The book was finished during my mother Beyhan Seckinelgin's unexpected illness and recovery during the spring of 2016 in Kuwait. Despite her condition, she was curious to learn about the book and keen to hear some of the discussion. Throughout this period, I was looked after very well and supported in my work. I thank my brother and his wife, Murat and Anna Tamer, for this. This book is also the outcome of an ongoing conversation throughout life with Damien Fennell. His support, encouragement and good humour have been essential ingredients in writing the book. As always, he has been my first reader, and his suggestions and interventions have helped me think and write clearly. His being there helps me live with contentment and happiness. The book is dedicated to him and to my mother who loves reading and loves books.

Contents

Chapter 1
Introduction

What interests me in this book is to consider the implications of the existing thinking on HIV intervention policies for the future. Currently, evaluation of success in the fight against HIV measures the present against the past by considering key milestones in the international struggle against HIV. Numerous international and national organizations have taken part in such evaluations.

One of the most comprehensive recent evaluations of the state of AIDS was developed by UNAIDS as part of the evaluation of the Millennium Development Goals in 2015. The document is entitled *How AIDS Changed Everything* (UNAIDS 2015a). Throughout its 545 pages, the report documents exhaustively what has been achieved in the struggle against HIV up to 2015. The report is comprehensive in its coverage of the field but also in its inclusion of relevant voices, including those of other international organizations and politicians and scientists leading debate within the field. In looking at progress in tackling HIV and AIDS the report states

> the global AIDS response continues to represent the most inspiring example of what can be achieved through international solidarity and evidence- and human rights –based action. Over more than three decades, the world has mounted a response to AIDS that serves as an inspiration for global health and international development… Ending the epidemic will demand not only the global community continues and builds on these gains, but also that the pace of scale-up is fast-tracked. In particular the AIDS response needs to accelerate progress in geographical settings and among populations where progress has not been shared equitably (2015a: 103).

In a similar way, the report seeks to provide insights into these gains. For instance it says,

> a comparison of the global distribution of antiretroviral therapy between 2000 and 2014 illustrates how profoundly the push towards universal treatment action has transformed the AIDS response. In 2000 2 % [2–3 %] of all people living with HIV were receiving antiretroviral therapy but 40 % [37–45 %] were receiving HIV treatment by 2014 (2015a: 109).

Furthermore, it is argued that

H. Seckinelgin, *The Politics of Global AIDS*, Social Aspects of HIV 3,
DOI 10.1007/978-3-319-46013-0_1

> [b]ased on available data it is projected that total amounts available for HIV programmes in low and middle income countries will reach US$ 21.7 billion in 2015. The total amount of resources invested for the AIDS response between 2000 and 2014 is estimated to be US$ 187.5 billion. Domestic investments by low and middle income countries have largely driven by the rise in HIV –related resources in recent years and this is likely to continue… The impact of these investments is notable. Between 2000 and 2014 over 7.8 million lives have been saved with antiretroviral therapy (2015a: 112).

These comparisons are just a small sample of the many that are contained within the volume. They show that principal mechanism behind these judgements involves highlighting where the issue was in the early 1980 alongside where we are today. The evaluation also follows the progressive development of policies targeting HIV during this period. The clear differences between 1980s and today, and the trajectory of these policy developments, provide an evaluation that shows how successful international actions have been in been changing the trends. It is clear from the extracts above that the language used to construct the Global AIDS response tells one of the most important success stories in the international arena.

However, the report also recognizes a number of problems that remain for the global response. These are presented in more cautious language than the language of success and solidarity used for the central themes underpinning the report. For instance, it is said that 'there are signs that stigma and discrimination may be declining as the HIV epidemic matures and more people with HIV live healthy lives thanks to antiretroviral therapy' (2015a: 114). This statement is supported by a review of the anti-discriminatory measures in place in a number of countries rather than the actual experiences of people with HIV. Another example of this caution is provided the statement that '[g]lobally, women account for 51 % of all adults living with HIV. Women represent 59 % of all people living with HIV in sub-Saharan Africa… Adolescent girls and young women are at especially high risk of acquiring HIV' (2015a: 100). Considering these statements in relation to the issues used to highlight the overall 'success' of the Global AIDS response, calls for a deeper analysis of the success story and the context within which it is articulated.

Crucially, these forms of evaluation of success pays little or no attention to the way in which the political process surrounding Global AIDS and the politics of solidarity have implications for the future. Any concern for the future seems to be framed, as shown above, within the limited horizon of the need to scale-up what we know works, and the need to maintain public solidarity on AIDS to facilitate the funding need to achieve this. Therefore, a document such as *How AIDS Changed Everything* constitutes not just an evaluation, but is also a strategy to establish the relevance of existing mechanisms for Global AIDS interventions of the future. While the success story is measured against the past, what this success story means for the future is not considered directly. In this book, my aim is to look more critically at this.

The analytic starting point for what follows lies in the future implications of a 'success story' based on the emergency model of response that has facilitated Global AIDS to date. The central issue I identify is that there is a need for a major shift from this emergency logic to a policy focus on wellbeing that is more broadly about the politics of the sustainability of lives.[1] This requires us also to think about how the fullness of peoples' overall lives may be linked to the policies and the politics of Global AIDS.[2]

By the term 'politics', I mean much more than just politics as actors negotiating or debating about various interests in order to gain access to resources. While this is, of course, part of the discussion, I want to consider how this process of politics has institutionalized certain ways of thinking and acting about HIV and AIDS through policy interventions within the field of AIDS as a global disease. In other words, my focus is on how the idea of Global AIDS has become a grounding position that guides thinking and acting in often quite different places. This way of thinking is clearly evident in a number of statements from eminent political actors given for the UNAIDS report mentioned above. For instance, in his response to interview questions Michel Sidibé, the executive director of UNAIDS, states that

> the last decade has been about scale-up, really massive scale-up and this could only happen with country leadership, community resilience and a shared vision of getting zero'. He then goes on to say that '[t]he AIDS movement is focused on reaching, protecting and promoting the rights of the most vulnerable…[w]e launched the Global Plan together with PEPFAR in 2011. We pushed countries with the highest burden to act. We mobilized the money (2015a: 23).

Here, in his words we have a basic mapping of actors and relations that are brought together under what is called the AIDS movement.[3] Through this framing, we gain a sense of global community and the 'AIDS movement' that comprises global activists and local actors in addition to international organizations and UNAIDS, as denoted by the use of the word 'we'. In addition, there is also in the report a portfolio of tools for advocacy and policy implementation that are used commonly across many different countries. The thinking that is created by this combination of factors is what I call the idea of *Global AIDS* that lies within this book.

The description of multi-layered relations, actors and activities identify the AIDS movement as the key agent for past change and success, built on a global solidarity as its base. At the same time, this description of success becomes the evidence for the political necessity of a Global AIDS framing for the future. Here, a success story 'ties together numerous experiences into a single term' (Koselleck 2002: 229). The single term here is that of 'Global AIDS', which comes to denote a global perspective and a shared understanding underpinned by global solidarity. The global

[1] One of the central issues raised about sustainability is about the sustainability of the treatment interventions over time (Shadlen 2013).

[2] My understanding of sustainability is broader than just particular Government's ability to maintain what has been done by the Global AIDS system (Pereira 2013). I consider sustainability as a political process which enables people to maintain their wellbeing. This no doubt needs engagement with governments among other actors but it requires more than lobbying to maintain the *status quo*. It is about having the ability to influence change as experiences of HIV and AIDS change in different contexts.

[3] The idea of AIDS movement makes sense according to Charles Tilly's definition of social movement. He considered social movements as having number of aspects. They have campaigns, repertoires of contention and Worthness, Unity, Numbers and Commitments (WUNC) (2004).

description of the movement that is implicit in the success narrative is also a political act. In order to understand the nature of the politics at work here, a careful unpacking of the institutionalized mechanisms of thinking about and acting on AIDS is needed. This unpacking is made possible by considering how both AIDS debate and the research underpinning this debate has come to look at the world through an 'AIDS lens', which brings together different experiences and issues to form Global AIDS debate. It is through this kind of analysis that one can begin to understand the implications of today's politics for the future.

In this introductory chapter, I first focus on the idea of politics which grounds my analytical approach to understand both the nature of Global AIDS and its implications. I then highlight through the analysis of one specific event the way in which Global AIDS is practised. The aim of this section to underline why I think there is a need to consider the politics of Global AIDS rather than the global politics of AIDS. Following this, I outline the methodological grounds that make the analysis of the politics of Global AIDS possible. I then conclude with an outline of the remainder of the book.

1.1 How to Think About Politics?

In this chapter, I want to look more closely at the idea of politics that is framing my analysis. In particular, I discuss a shift from the politics of organizational bargaining towards a notion of politics as practice that acts to create a particular way of thinking about a subject. This discussion is important, as it is often not very clear what is meant by the politics of AIDS. My approach, by considering politics as practice, focuses on how to identify this politics I would like to analyse, and also the spaces *wherein which we find this politics.*

To start with, I want to consider the politics of AIDS as it has emerged in the last three decades as a politics of solidarity. This kind of politics has generated an understanding of Global AIDS as a humanitarian emergency requiring the attention of an AIDS movement.[4] In thinking about solidarity and the way in which it has been made so central to the politics of AIDS, I want to consider solidarity as a process of soliciting support and then disciplining this support to achieve a common target, which is projected as being in everyone's interest. Because of this, thinking about the politics of AIDS requires considering how such politics of solidarity can be maintained over time in the changing circumstances in which people live with HIV. In other words, our interest has to be in how the politics of solidarity is reproduced in general, and what its impact is on new circumstances based on the politics of wellbeing and the politics of recognition and redistribution within a particular context. To be clear, I want to observe the politics of the AIDS movement as a

[4] Here, the issue is the way in which AIDS is framed as a problem that needs global attention to locate it as a policy concern in competition with other problems in various contexts, both nationally and internationally (see Hoppe 2011: 2–8).

political practice that needs to maintain solidarity in order to legitimate its agency, but which at the same time also needs to transform itself without losing this agency. This tension raises questions about the nature and limits of solidarity as it has emerged as an emergency response. It also highlights the way in which this solidarity has been solidified as a structural mechanism that governs the future of people's wellbeing within particular contexts.

This view of politics is inspired by Jacques Rancière's reflections on politics 'as a mode of practice by a specific kind of subject and deriving from a particular kind of reason' (2010: 27). The claim here is twofold: (a) the politics of AIDS forms a particular mode of practice and then, (b) this mode of practice creates a particular kind of subject. Through this way of thinking about politics, it is possible to disentangle politics as *a mode of practice* from a meta-understanding of politics 'as the exercise of power' (Rancière 2010: 27). Such a move allows analysis to shift from a limited understanding of politics as an approach to the evaluation of organizational practices and their grounds, to a focus on the exercise of power, which is more interested in how those organizational practices are created in the first place (Rancière 2010: 27). While the former approach is concerned with modalities of governance (see Parker 2002; Paxton 2012), it overlooks the way in which politics as practice is productive. In the former approach, the ideal form of good governance is taken as a central way to achieve the political good for those who are part of the organizational system (see Strand 2012). The global politics of AIDS considered in this way is about the analysis of the role played by various actors in organizational negotiations and bargaining aimed at generating and allocating resources for particular AIDS-related interventions. This organizational approach focuses on how within these processes certain policy outcomes are created at multiple levels of decision making and implementation. Much of the research from this organizational position focuses on how various organizations – that include intergovernmental organizations, funding agencies, non-governmental organizations – and their interests produce effective policies, or how different actors need to coordinate their work to address the problems created by HIV and AIDS in different countries across the globe (Pereira 2013; Siplon 2013; Patten et al. 2013). Here, the globe comes to mean the geographically comprehensive reach of international processes. The focus becomes the appropriateness and development of particular policy tools related to governance mechanisms for dealing with the problem of HIV and AIDS in multiple contexts. Within such a vision, concerns about delivery and considerations of political leadership take prominence as the main issues for analysis. An analysis of the global politics of AIDS thereby becomes largely concerned with the emergence and development of the international organizations that have developed global knowledge, policy and implementation competence on HIV by leading global advocacy work on AIDS. I want to argue, however, that this approach positions itself within already existing AIDS debate. Analyses are limited to concerns over organizational effectiveness, often framed as 'efficiency' in policy development, the delivery of resources or their distribution among designated target groups. Such an approach no doubt has its merits and still remains relevant.[5] However, it is also limited in its understanding of the impacts of what might be considered to be the global politics of AIDS on HIV and AIDS in different contexts.

The move I am making here considers politics as a particular practice that creates Global AIDS as a particular problem within which subjects and subjectivities are produced and reproduced. This is to provide an alternative lens to introverted discussions and evaluations of politics that gradually homogenise subjects and their needs, and which determine their relations to each other and the way in which they should partake 'in being ruled' (Rancière 2010: 27). This differentiation is important as it signifies a separation between understanding politics as correct forms of governing in general, and understanding politics as a practice in which subjects participate on the basis of 'private or domestic world of needs or interests' to challenge the modalities of good governance to supply them with good policies (Rancière 2010: 36). The idea of politics cast in this latter way allows for the possibility of understanding how the idea and subject of Global AIDS have emerged and changed. It also reveals how this framing once formed, further frames the practices of Global AIDS. In other words, it leads us to an understand how in this process different ways of being and acting in a common world are created by Global AIDS to address the problem of AIDS.

In this alternative approach, the idea of partaking in the practice of politics provides the central analytical grounding. It offers us a lens through which to consider the possibility of, or limits of, partaking and the conditions that determine such processes. Politics here then is about the relations that are determined by this dynamic process. Rancière's thinking offers a mode of understanding the way in which subjects, based on their needs, partake in challenging their subjectification by organizational forms. This allows us to think in a new way about the practice of politics. In contrast, a more conventional organizational approach ignores this process of partaking, as it presents a challenge to the organizational realm by people who are presenting their own subject positions. According to Rancière, '[p]olitics disappears the moment you undo this knot of a subject and a relation' (2010: 29). Politics, in his view, emerges in constant attempts to define subjects and challenges to these descriptions based on located domestic needs and interests. Such a perspective rejects a view of politics that limits itself to attempts to describe subjects within larger organizational processes as reductive. It rejects also the idea of ready-made subject categories, such as citizen, and of the particular kinds of organizational form that are considered to be relevant political domain for politics. In other words, it embraces the challenge of dynamic everyday life.

In this approach to politics, Rancière is concerned primarily with the dominant views that homogenise the subject of politics. He argues that

[5]An interesting example of this is the important work by Lesley and Len Doyal (2013). My approach to politics is an attempt to take their argument further to identify the mechanisms as to why things remain unanswered in the system independent of policy campaigns and statements to include people's needs.

> [p]olitics is commonly viewed as the practice of power or the embodiment of collective wills and interests and enactment of collective ideas…imply that you are taken into account as subjects sharing things located in a common world…what really deserves the name of politics is the cluster of perceptions and practices that shape this common world (2010: 152).

He considers the politics of consensus as a way of homogenising voices to create ideal communities. As a corollary, I argue that the conventional analysis based on a limited organizational understanding of politics also ignores the challenges of partaking and ways in which these challenges create different subject positions within a political process. Rancière argues that 'the essence of politics [then] is to disturb this arrangement by supplementing it with a part of the no-part identified with the community as a whole' (2010: 36). The point here is that the politics that aims to form an ideal community will always be based on designating at the same time those who are *not* to take part – the no-part of it – or those who will disappear from this kind of politics. So, his approach argues that

> Politics is first of all a way of framing, among sensory data, a specific sphere of experience. It is a partition of the sensible, of the visible, and the sayable, which allows (or does not allow) some specific data to appear; which allows or does not allow some specific subjects to designate them and speak about them (Rancière 2010: 152)

and that thereby '[p]olitics is first and foremost an intervention upon the visible and the sayable' (Rancière 2010: 152). His approach is more to think about politics as *dissensus* when he argues that 'the essence of politics resides in the modes of dissensual subjectification that reveal the difference of a society to itself' (Rancière 2010: 38). In this, he defines the social not as 'a particular sphere of existence but, rather, a disputed object of politics' (Rancière 2010: 43).

Given the civil society activism that grounds the global AIDS movement, and the way in which the AIDS has become both national and international public policy concern, Rancière's position on politics as partaking in a process of subjectification, provides an appropriate lens through which to consider the politics of Global AIDS. The way in which the politics of solidarity emerged around AIDS suggests a political process in which the 'voiceless' have indeed provided alternative voices. These were based on their needs and interests within the broader community, initially from within particular national contexts and then gradually more internationally. Rancière's view allows analysis to focus on a politics of AIDS that is revealed in the dynamic intersections of attempts to limit partaking and challenges to these attempts to influence social change. In this way, my analysis will focus (a) on the nature of politics of solidarity on AIDS as it has emerged and (b) the way in which this politics of solidarity in turn evolved into a global solidarity politics. In other words, as the politics of partaking challenges top-down subjectification and provides a dynamic lens through which to consider internal change within the AIDS movement, the lens of politics as partaking provides a number of avenues to explore: (a) the way in which emerging solidarity around AIDS challenged political authority in its early years, (b) the way in which this politics of solidarity underpinned the internationalization of the politics of AIDS, and (c) how the internationalization of concern for AIDS has created its own patterns of subjectification as a political practice. Consideration of these pathways is central to understand the politics of AIDS today, or what I call in this book Global AIDS, and its implications for the future.

1.2 An Audience in the Court of Global AIDS

In addressing a gathered multi-disciplinary social scientists working on HIV at the pre-conference workshop entitled *Ensuring a Supportive Environment for Effective Long-term HIV Response: Social and political challenges* on 20 July 2012, which took place just before 2012 International AIDS conference in Washington DC, the then executive director of International AIDS Society (IAS) began his talk by thanking scholars for their participation in the workshop. He emphasized the importance given to the social sciences and their contributions to the global AIDS response by IAS and the AIDS world it represents. One of the issues he highlighted was the way in which social sciences can still help to think about behaviour and the context of behaviour change, as well as to provide pathways for dealing with the consequences of changes in the international aid regime. After this positive, but generic statement, he went on to argue however that in the end *HIV* 'is a medical condition and that we expect the advances in this area will have the biggest impact on the disease. In this, undoubtedly the social sciences can be helpful but they are not going to have the same impact in dealing with HIV'. According to his position this has important implications for thinking about social science response to HIV. Given the primary framing of HIV as a medical condition and the importance of medical solutions in dealing with it, the social sciences, so the audience was told, will have to make sure that their added value is clear as part of a broader response. Given limited resources for research, the preferred option was to choose the aspects of social science research that best support broader developments emerging from the medical sciences. Clearly, the speaker was not interested in thinking comprehensively about a social science approach to HIV and AIDS.

This was a seriously uncomfortable situation for those of us in the audience. After spending a day and a half discussing socio-political challenges in the response to AIDS and how to establish a comprehensive research agenda on HIV from within the social sciences, the audience was told how the Global AIDS community felt about the role of social sciences. Many in the audience were not impressed. Their main reaction was to consider this situation as yet another reflection of the biomedical, technical, framing of HIV in which social sciences have but a marginal role. This is a reasonable interpretation. However, as much as the content of the speech, the way in which the speech was delivered was also important. Thinking about this particular event over time, I have come to realize that what happened was not simply the result of two different scientific framings of HIV and the way in which the tension between them informed the executive-director's position. The issue was about how the framing of the disease has come to be, and how this has been deployed time and again to reproduce a particular position and a horizon towards which everyone is to be directed within the international AIDS community. This speech, this way of speaking, was more a delineation, an ordering, an exercise in which the nature of the problem was once more reiterated and the assumed agency of different actors, including scientists, was highlighted. This setting out of the terrain was also a way of establishing how *we* should plan and manage our response to AIDS. Importantly, the idea of the 'we' here was reiterated by emphasizing the strength of the community engaging with AIDS in solidarity with each other. Thus, the existence of the self-identified AIDS community and its global nature were reproduced.

This approach to understanding the nature of HIV presents AIDS as the biomedically defined target against which 'we' are all fighting. Through this unifying approach, we all are incorporated into a Global AIDS framing. While social scientists are relevant in this debate, they are not there to critically discuss and re-think ongoing global AIDS interventions and the new challenges the epidemic poses. Here, in his way of speaking, the then executive director of the IAS was reproducing the idea of the Global AIDS context, derived from setting AIDS as a unified target. He set out what 'really matters' in facing the AIDS challenge, reiterating the nature of the problem as a medical and technical condition. This, was intended to guide us, the audience, as members of the larger AIDS community, to think more carefully about AIDS and how to plan to tackle it. This position, from within Global AIDS, brooks no criticism and does not allow for engagement that might challenge the framing of AIDS as a global disease.

This ordering, or guiding, speech was also a way of reiterating the other important component of the Global AIDS framing, namely the supposed 'solidarity' of the AIDS movement across the globe. Considering the civil society and activist background of the then IAS executive director, his position also implicitly grounded this Global AIDS view as an understanding of the broader solidarity. The speech sought to elicit a pact with the audience to be together within this Global AIDS framing. The speech was important in its setting out the priorities for Global AIDS thinking while also trying to sustain the solidaristic outlook without which the idea of Global AIDS cannot be sustained. This double movement, to assert a particular understanding of AIDS based on specific knowledge claims and to project a unity of purpose – solidarity – in the face of AIDS everywhere, also reinforces thinking about the disease within a global framing. The meta-framing of AIDS as medico-technical problem allows AIDS to be set apart as a global object of interest. From this, everyone who is interested in this object becomes part of the solidarity, which in turn underlines the idea of its global character. This homogenizes and links a multiplicity of experiences, needs and the required differentiated knowledge to understand these into a general debate under the Global AIDS rubric. The idea of solidarity in the face of the common objective is the mechanism through which the technical process of dealing with the disease can be operationalized and maintained as part of a global approach.

While this largely technical description of the problem creates an uniform and objectified target, it is not enough to support a framing that is comprehensive in its claims to order, to plan and to manage AIDS debate *globally*. Operationalizing the medico-technical logic of targeting in multiple contexts rests also on the ability to incorporate other actors and to maintain their participation in this process. The idea of 'solidarity' provides the grounds on which this incorporation is managed and maintained. This idea, first, establishes an attitude towards others. It begins by identifying people who are exposed to the same problem. The technical description of similarity and knowledge claims underwriting the technical know-how allows the articulation of a responsibility to act on the problem to help these people. Thus, the scope of discussion is expanded. Moreover, by identifying a similarity based on exposure to a shared problem, different actors are brought into the solidarity network. Via this process, solidarity from a particular lens – in this case AIDS – is used to construct lives and narratives from a particular vantage point, which I have called elsewhere, 'communities of policy as opposed to the communities of everyday life' (Seckinelgin 2012a).

The politics that I am interested in this book therefore is not only about the way in which this Global AIDS framing has been created and reproduced, but also its impact on the future of HIV-related intervention in everyday lives. There is no doubt that questions about the relevance of my approach can be raised from within the Global AIDS fora. An immediate critical issue would be about whether this approach serves as a diversion from *our* work to fight AIDS. It could be argued that the approach does not provide *us* with the new tools needed to tackle the AIDS problem across the world. However, as relevant as these questions may appear, they are inherently located within the Global AIDS debate itself, and its self-production processes. Indeed, they are produced through the double movement I outline above: *in solidarity to tackle a ('our') common technical objective*. They frame the relevance of research or discussions according to their immediate perceived utility to deal with the AIDS problem as identified by the Global AIDS framing, and are therefore subject to the limitations of this approach.

An objection could also be raised on the grounds that the technical objectification of AIDS as uniform issue globally has in fact produced good results. Many AIDS-related policy developments are based on technical knowledge of HIV and methods of interventions e.g. from the use of condoms to the development of antiretroviral treatment to voluntary medical male circumcision and the emergence of pre-exposure prophylaxis as methods of prevention. However, in the idea of tackling Global AIDS in an unified manner, what is to be targeted by these methods is also viewed uniformly. In other words, Global AIDS, through its thinking about the supply of policies and implementation tools, homogenizes audiences and target groups. This leads to marginalization and perhaps the eventual disappearance of demand side claims for different kinds of policy thinking. This approach focuses advocacy work on AIDS broadly on questions of the availability of these means of intervention across the globe, and access to them by those who are in need. In this sense, a Global AIDS framing is about increasing equal access to the resources that are available to deal with AIDS at the time of an emergency.

The evaluation of these outcomes, in many cases as successful outcomes, is discussed in *How AIDS Changed Everything* (UNAIDS 2015a). However, this evaluation has very little to say about future implications and possibilities. Considered from this perceptive, I argue that on the one hand some of these outcomes are important and in comparison with the past they do show improved state of affairs. On the other hand, however, their evaluation also hides major disparities between different groups as briefly mentioned above, for instance in relation to women, on issues of stigma and discrimination, and particularly discrimination directly against sexual and gender minorities. Furthermore, such evaluations limit the discussions for future on ideas around scaling-up by not reflecting on the conditions of sustainability for many of the interventions that underwrite present success narratives. They focus on improved technical ability to deliver new products rather than questions of how to maintain people's wellbeing over time beyond having access to what are framed as essential tools to fight HIV within the dominant framings offered by Global AIDS. Peoples' wellbeing is narrowly considered. Rather than looking at matters from the point of view of those people targeted, the possibility of such access is considered to be about maintaining the global solidarity that has produced the successful results that were identified in the first place.

1.3 How Then to Approach Global AIDS?

The politics of Global AIDS frames much current international debate and supports itself by reiterating its relevance to its global community and to the solidarity needed to fight HIV. This process of reproducing a particular view, which at the same time attempting to introduce change, requires us to fully understand the mechanisms that make this possible. This requires a methodological approach that allows one to think about mechanisms of reproduction and change that also maintains a sense of community. This is a dynamic process with its own 'quality controls and the allowance and disallowance of information, procedural and competence rules for who can and cannot participate in the question-and-answer game' (Hoppe 2011: 4).

As I mentioned above, within Global AIDS framework research and discussions are often evaluated according to how they fit with particular tendencies within this framework at a given period. For instance, one very experienced colleague, who was very much involved with UNAIDS from its early days and who has since become in international expert advising on many aspects of global AIDS policy, would often in her evaluation of research include a statement about how a given research would be appropriate, or not, according to *international policy priorities* and *accepted knowledge claims* in international fora. This is an interesting example of how research evaluation may also act as a disciplining process that ensures the reproduction of a common framework. In her advisory work, this same person would take international agreed policy statements as the boundaries of the policy direction within which a given research needed to be located. This approach to evaluation delineates what 'matters' from what does not within a global AIDS framework, recognising and delineating the boundaries of Global AIDS. However, it does not consider the way in which international policy priorities are set and their limitations, or allow for a direct questioning of these priories or the knowledge claims that justify them. Indeed, this position perpetuates a tension between working together in an overall project to fight AIDS globally and the freedom to engage critically with the governance of policies targeting AIDS. This is a productive tension because it disciplines researchers to position their questions first within existing policy priorities so that they can be considered relevant to ongoing discussion and second, to underline their commitment to the wider and supposedly 'shared' goals of the community. While no doubt this creates a research approach that focuses minds and effort, it also leaves many critical issues and questions outside this *virtuous circle* of solidarity.

Up until recently, this position was also supported as mentioned above by the emergency logic of fighting AIDS, which had framed most international thinking. At times of an emergency, one has to deal with the immediate issues, *critical engagements questioning the direction of travel are not relevant at this stage*. One has often heard that *we don't have time for this now we have to deal with the immediate needs.* This is a strong boundary regulation that establishes what may be seen as the relevant and allowed in an emergency context. Furthermore, it creates a relationship that encourages researchers to participate in a collective move towards dealing with the emergency. The methodological issue here is about how research becomes self-referential with in the Global AIDS framework as a result of these emergency imperatives and the need to show solidarity with Global AIDS horizons. Again, some may argue that such a claim is too strong and does not acknowledge internal discussions within Global AIDS on policy options and knowledge claims. I disagree. There is no doubt that there is a diversity of voices and positions that challenge each other within the global AIDS community. However, these challenges are then resolved by a meta-appeal to a particular policy direction according to priorities underwritten by a set of particularly privileged knowledge claims and the emergency logic that legitimizes the approach on humanitarian grounds. The example I used earlier in the form of the speech by the then IAS executive-director, provides one such illustration of this. It allows for an internal diversity of voices but this diversity *must be channelled* in a way of acting that fits a set of priorities already determined by elite actors. If this does not work, the spirit of solidarity as leverage is always the next strategy to be deployed to bring everyone into line. Similarly, people may argue that the emergency logic does not apply anymore as UNAIDS has clearly moved from this position as evidenced by number of recent statements (see for instance UNAIDS 2015b). This is correct. However, for people living with HIV, the problem remains. This move does not allow critical questioning of either the implications of having a system created in an emergency mode or of the future implications of this rather late acknowledgement by UNAIDS and others that HIV needs to be considered from a different lens – one more in line with the global Sustainable Development Goals (SDGs) (UNAIDS and Lancet Commission 2015; UNAIDS 2016a). That said, this recent move only changes the way policy language frames the focus of the debate; control over the nature of this debate, which the AIDS community should be having, is maintained.

The brief analysis above reveals a set of relations within Global AIDS that have evolved into a coherent set of practices, comprising a relatively homogeneous system for thinking and acting. In this way, Global AIDS allows engagement with HIV that produces particular ways of being and acting. It also shows that these relations are broadly patterned through communication processes that include knowledge production practices in the form of published documents and policy announcements, as well as in events like workshops and conferences, but also research evaluations and dissemination processes. These communication processes become boundary control mechanisms that maintain the ways in which the system changes in a self-referential manner. These changes highlight the fact that when we are talking about the Global AIDS framework, our concern is with an internal system of priority setting, knowledge production, creation of policy directions and evaluation of strategies. Policy implementation is then evaluated according to these priorities so as to be able to account for success (Hoppe 2011: 130–142). This is reflected in policy assessments as they reflect the internally set priorities and monitored procedures. The document I mentioned earlier, *How AIDS Changed Everything,* and others published in the same vein establish a common history for Global AIDS-to establish common ground (UNAIDS 2015d, e, UNAIDS 2016b). As Kosseleck argues, 'various ways of narrating histories or processing them methodologically can be related to the ways in which experiences are made, collected or transformed' (2002: 50). Applied to HIV, these strategies are also about AIDS organizations partaking 'in the stabilization of given experiences' (Kosseleck 2002: 52). Furthermore, creating a common history legitimates particular ways of knowing as most claims on policy success are justified from within particular ways of thinking about policy relevant research for Global AIDS. As tools for communicating both within the AIDS community and with its wider environment, the common narrative sets the record and the assumptions that guide future direction for new generations of people who would like to work in this field.

Such an internal process requires an external environment against which internal mechanisms are set, maintained and reproduced. The external environment here includes the broader international policy fields of health, international development, education and other fields, such as those identified in the Millennium Development Goals. The relationship between Global AIDS as a system and its environment is based on drawing distinctions to designate what matters for the system in its engagement with the environment. One of the key main ideas that allows this process to work is the idea of AIDS as an emergency policy concern. This has created a zone of exception within the broader policy context to focus attention on AIDS in competition with other problems (McFalls 2010). The other central idea that grounds this process of differentiation lies in the view of Global AIDS as a system of solidarity. The importance of communicating this sense of solidarity internally matters as much as it does externally, since it motivates actors to support it in the times of an emergency. As a result, it is possible to observe the politics of Global AIDS in the boundary control mechanisms that are often employed within policy discussions and in the language used in discussions about HIV. However, to think more politically about AIDS, in the way I frame the idea of the politics, is challenging.

As someone who has worked on HIV, and as someone who has been part of the Global AIDS process for many years, can I step out of this dominant framing to analyse it? How do we analyze these circumstances and disciplined change politically without being forced into the boundaries of the discussion? This requires thinking about Global AIDS from a methodologically innovative position. According to Niklas Luhmann 'the operation of social communication produces the unity of the social system by recursively referring back and forward to other social communication, creating a *distinction* between system and environment'(1998: 18). What matters in this process is the way in which the idea of solidarity in the face of an emergency is communicated so as both to frame the system and to legitimate particular actors' agency to speak on behalf of Global AIDS. Here Luhmann's articulation provides another layer for analysis. He suggests that the language choices that are made to distinguish the system, also act internally to maintain and delineate the internal understanding of the system. He argues that the system 'distinguishes itself by the execution of the *observation*, which must distinguish this communication from others or the environment from systems that are reproduced through this operation. Observation must and can choose distinctions' (1998: 18). Once observation is considered from this angle, as a language that is chosen, that is as a practice which is operationalized as a systemic boundary mechanism, it becomes possible to consider the content of observation to understand the operations of the system: what is reproduced as a relationship within the system and in its relationship to its environment. Luhmann suggests that the system 'can be observed with regard to the distinctions that it chooses or avoids choosing' (1998: 18). It is in these choices and what these choices include or exclude, that the politics of Global AIDS can be critically analyzed.

According to Luhmann,

> observation means nothing more than handling distinctions… self-observation is the introduction of the system/environment distinction within the system, which constitutes itself with the help of that distinction; … for elements to be reproduced, it must be guaranteed that they are reproduced as elements of the system and not as anything else (Luhmann 1998: 36–37).

In this sense, the possibility of analyzing the system that I have called Global AIDS, rests with observing this self-production process. In Luhmann's terms, this is called 'secondary observation' (1998: 47–62). He argues that these kinds of observations

> are observations of observations. This can include observations of other observers or observations of the same or different actors at different points in time. Depending on these variants, social and temporal dimensions can be distinguished in the production of meaning (1998: 48).

This position is important as it allows, in line with the framing of politics I discussed above, a move from self-analysis within the system geared towards maintaining a general consensual systemic understanding, to more contingent ways of thinking about the way the system develops and works. In particular, it allows us to observe the operationalization of particular ways of thinking about a subject, in this case HIV and AIDS. This also ties to how best to think about the contingency issue. According to Luhmann, in first-level self-observation the observer 'constitutes the distinction by designating, by going from "unmarked space" to "marked space".

And what is designated is itself directly present in the execution of the observation operation' (1998: 47). Therefore self-observation does not account for the contingency of its own operation, of its reproduction. For instance, the standard questions that could be raised, mentioned above, concerning critical enquiries on AIDS are part of this self-observation of Global AIDS maintained through the evaluation and monitoring of research, policies and implementation. In a similar way, discussion of the politics that limits debate to organizational improvements and good governance for better HIV-related policy functions to reproduce the systemic view and does not allow for observations of the overall operational system. Even when new organizations are created, they are created within the self-understandings of the latter.

The methodology of secondary observation as an analytical tool provides an alternative angle from which to evaluate the impact of the Global AIDS interventions I discussed earlier. The nature of evaluation in this particular instance is interesting as it produces a history of the Global AIDS phenomenon that then establishes its relevance *as the* framework with which to deal with people's problems in relation to HIV in the future. This methodological orientation focuses attention on the way in which actors talk about AIDS and what has been achieved over time. The analysis pays special attention to how these discussions reproduce Global AIDS. The value of this approach is that one does not need to leave the Global AIDS debate and externalize oneself to it to be able to analyse it. It offers entry points to focus the analysis on how the system creates functional differentiation for its practice within a particular environment, and how it communicates these differentiations within its practice over time. It therefore introduces a time factor into the analysis with which to consider the change and the institutionalization which needs to reproduce itself.

1.4 The Book

The book is divided into six chapters and a concluding chapter that provides an alternative view on how to think about evaluation of success in this field. The first three chapters focus on the development of politics of solidarity on AIDS and its transformation into the politics of Global AIDS. The following three chapters then focus on the ways in which the Global AIDS framing impacts on knowledge production and claims of policy relevance, and how these in turn come to reassert the relevance of a Global AIDS perspective for future dealing with the epidemic. Throughout these chapters, I aim to provide a distinct and distinctive challenge to *How AIDS Changed Everything's* claim that 'the global AIDS response continues to represent the most inspiring example of what can be achieved through international solidarity and evidence – and human rights-based action'(UNAIDS 2015a: 103). In this way, the structural limitations of the system in responding to people's changing wellbeing needs can be unpacked.

Chapter 2
Pathways to the Politics of Global AIDS and the Meanings of AIDS

This chapter looks at the emergence of the politics of Global AIDS by considering the multiple social and political challenges that have been confronted and responded to by different actors. This is important, as it highlights some of the key factors influencing the meanings of AIDS and Global AIDS today. David Caron's reflection on being HIV positive provides an important entry point to these issues when he states that

> … one is not HIV positive in a cultural and political vacuum. In fact, there is no other experience of HIV than one that is saturated with politics and culture. That's why it's so messy and so slippery, so dynamic that it can never sit still long enough to constitute a stable object of knowledge (Caron 2014:24).

Central here is the claim that the way in which HIV is apprehended depends on the circumstances. Contextual factors create particular understandings of the disease, which evolve as circumstances change. I argue that a similar process also applies to the way in which the politics of AIDS developed throughout the 1980s and 1990s in the pre-1996 period prior to the creation of UNAIDS. In a similar way to how people with HIV had to make sense of a new disease, so too did organizations, both nationally and internationally, as they engaged with the emergence of a new disease within specific socio-political circumstances.[1] The different ways in which AIDS was understood often led to competing meanings of the disease. This chapter provides an analysis of some of these processes and the politics that accompanied them.

In the course of these events it is not only possible to observes the sources of information and the qualities that came to frame AIDS, but also how gradually a shared global understanding of the disease began to emerge. Crucially, this process

[1] By political circumstances, I mean the political circumstances in which AIDS emerged as a new issue. One key factor influencing the politics of AIDS was the gay rights movement and related welfare discussions, particularly in the USA. Another factor was the environment within which international development policies were developed and implemented, as these influenced the funding available for particular issues.

H. Seckinelgin, *The Politics of Global AIDS*, Social Aspects of HIV 3,
DOI 10.1007/978-3-319-46013-0_2

of apprehending and then using what was apprehended to engage with others, constitutes the politics of AIDS. In an environment where there are competing apprehensions, reflecting different understandings of the disease, interactions between these different perspectives create a politics of contestation with respect to what it is that is being represented. This framing of politics differs from more conventional approaches to the political, which focus for example on what states do and/or what international organizations do. The framing I use here is also interested in what these actors do. However, it is also focused on *why* do they do what they do. This requires us to understand how different actors came to engage with and understand AIDS, the different meanings that derived from their experiences, and the way in which contestations between these created the basis of a politics.

This approach is in line with the definition of politics I set out in the previous chapter. In order to understand Global AIDS, we need to consider the dynamics and relations that motivate interactions between people with HIV, medical scientists, governments, international organizations and civil society groups. The contestations between these groups that I will describe are based on ways of being and thinking that lead to disagreement, which cause groups to negotiate for access to resources, which change the nature of bargaining by having a seat in a meeting, or that simply have to be taken into account when policy decisions take place. Politics in this sense, following Rancière, is about the activist 'who argues for the public nature of a "domestic" matter' and who 'must indicate the world in which his argument counts as an argument and must demonstrate it as such for those who do not possess a frame of reference to conceive of it as argument' (2010).

Throughout this chapter, I want to use this way of thinking about the 'domestic' to highlight how HIV as a personal experience transformed HIV into a public concern, providing new ways of thinking about the epidemic for the public at large. The logical extension of this argument is about how specific sets of meanings become internalized within different organizational/public domains. My argument is that actors act and react according to an internal set of understandings developed in the course of their everyday lives. These internalized meanings and actions generate particular relations and particular ways of managing the relations between different groups of actors. By examining the framing of AIDS as a global disease and by thinking about global politics, we are not only looking at organizational debates and discrete political actors, but also at multi-layered processes of negotiation, challenge and bargaining that highlight how different practices emerge in different contexts.

This perspective on politics focuses in on the different layers of disagreement about AIDS, and the negotiations between them throughout the 1980s and the early 1990s. My analysis aims to highlight how these disagreements institutionalized certain ways of thinking about AIDS. If we consider politics as a partaking that unpacks disagreements within society, the experience of AIDS in the USA and Western Europe in the 1980s and in the 1990s offers an entry point for understanding the politics of AIDS as it later emerged. At the same time, looking at similar interactions within the international arena highlights different aspects of the emergent Global AIDS.

2.1 Early Years

Although based on a broadly conventional analysis of international organizations, Leon Gordenker, Roger A. Coate, Christer Jönsson and Peter Söderholm's book *International Cooperation in Response to AIDS,* first published in 1995, is an important book for various reasons. First, it was ahead of its time as it looked at the international system from an AIDS lens and by doing so provided an innovative perspective from within the field of international relations. Second, the book provides insight into the conflicting mandates, policy interests and concerns within the international organizational context of the 1980s and the 1990s. As such, it provides a valuable micro-analysis of negotiations within and between various organizations. Perhaps most importantly, however, it is a historical document that enables us to understand a period of time, which has been to a degree lost from public discussion.

Franklyn Lisk's 2010 book *Global Institutions and the HIV/AIDS Epidemic* also offers an analysis of international organizations' responses to HIV and AIDS. To a degree it updates the earlier volume's discussion by providing insights into the creation of the UNAIDS. Given the availability of these sources, my analyses will not repeat what they outline as the genesis narrative for the emergence of AIDS as an international policy concern. However, I will consider their narratives to develop my analysis of the politics of AIDS as it emerged in the early 1990s. My aim here is not to be limited to a factual narrative of events but to reflect on the kind of politics that emerged from these events as a result of the challenges and disagreements that underwrote them, and the changes they signified for the politics of Global AIDS today.

It is clear that political questions around AIDS were already part of public debate at the time the disease first emerged. In their analysis, Gordenker et al. describe the international politics of AIDS at the time as follows

> ...... the pandemic will eventually reach very inhabited space of the earth. Surely this was an issue that clearly had global dimensions and required the cooperation of all authorities that could ordain responses to a pandemic. Either rational analysis or the application of influence by a dominant authority- in this case it would have to be a government- might have been expected to dictate a global response. Over the last decade, neither this kind of cooperation among governing agencies nor the domination of any government has appeared. Rather transnational cooperation...had a shifting, variable character and a variety of different organizations operated with a wide spectrum of approaches and techniques. ...A variety of organizational and personal goals- some constant, some vacillating, some implicit, some unstated-underlie their activity. Governments and their organizational components stand out in international cooperation on AIDS as a – but not the- principal source of information and resources, as well as the objects of agents of persuasion for others. That could not be otherwise in a world where public policy is formally adopted and in fact in large part supervised and administered through governmental apparatus. Governmental personnel constantly propose and often decide in the world of transnational cooperation. But the notion of a government acting as a unit would overlook the importance of its subunits developing their own transnational cooperative arrangements, both with opposite numbers in other governments and IGOs and their parts and with NGOs. Nor did the subunits of any one government continually dominate the scene (1995:135–136).

This extract outlines a situation that was to change fairly dramatically not too long after the publication of the book in 1995, both in terms of the way AIDS was tackled and with respect to international cooperation. Their analysis reveals however that different actors had different ideas and approaches, and were creating networks that they thought were good for them to achieve their ends. In this way, the field was seen as populated by largely uncoordinated actors and ideas trying to get something done about AIDS. While antiretroviral treatment turned HIV into a more or less manageable disease in resource-rich settings, the emergence of an international 'coordinating' body in the form of the Joint United National Programme on HIV and AIDS (UNAIDS), alongside this treatment, created the momentum to think in a more global way about the disease and the policies targeting it. Together, these changes provided a historical turning point for the politics of the disease both nationally and internationally. Prior to this, the response had been at best patchy. Local responses had been articulated by different actors, including non-governmental actors, but in the end coordination between various actors and their activities was weak. The global scope implicit in this argument concerns the geographic spread of the disease and international cooperation; thus the politics seems mostly to be about the internal work within the international organizations.

Lisk's work looking at the same period also frames the discussion in a similar way. Both books provide insight from a formal political organizational lens. They bring out some of the many challenges at both formal governmental and international organizational levels on how to deal with AIDS, how to develop responses to it, and how to coordinate these responses across countries and across international organizations. The politics of AIDS at the time was created by an attempt to overcome these challenges. Different actors wanted to engage differently based on their existing ways of dealing with this new condition and their organizational mandates. The engagement of different actors that included people living with AIDS, scientists, politicians, civil society organizations and formal local or international organizations across these mandates created a move towards thinking about AIDS as a common target for everyone, which in turn laid the foundations for Global AIDS.

A quick glance at several of the earlier reports by the United States' Centers for Disease Control (CDC) highlights a number of challenges to this newly observed condition. It was not known for sure what the cause of AIDS was until late 1983, so in many early reports concerns about the blood supply and about the best way to think about prevention figure strongly. Although reports at the time were written in a technical manner, the socio-political aspects of the situation were clear. Scientists and policy makers were struggling to find the risk factors and to identify the groups that were most at risk.

In June 1981, the CDC in its weekly Morbidity and Mortality Weekly Report (MMWR) reported the unexpected death of five patients from Los Angeles. After providing a short report on each patient, MMWR in its editorial note stated that all five had been diagnosed with '*Pneumocystis* pneumonia' adding that '*Pneumocystis* pneumonia in the United States is almost exclusively limited to severely immune suppressed patients' (1981). After pointing out that there was no obvious clinical reason for these deaths, the note states that '[t]he fact that these patients were all homosexuals suggests an association between some aspect of a homosexual lifestyle or disease acquired through sexual contact and *Pneumocystis* pneumonia in this population' (1981: 1). The nature of this observation located the disease issue in a context that was already charged with sexuality rights issues and political activism. Actions to demedicalize homosexuality constituted one of the main foci for ongoing struggles for sexuality rights at that point in time (Altman 1971). It was only in 1973 that the American Psychological Association removed homosexuality from its list of disorders and WHO maintained it in its list of disorders until 1992. This initial CDC positioning was therefore to have a major impact on the way the disease became a major public debate and concern.[2] Importantly, 1983 the Council of Europe issued a statement 'calling on the WHO to delete homosexuality from its International Classification of Diseases' (Gordenker et al. 1995:39). The Council was to issue further statements in 1983 and 1985 warning against the 'anti-homosexuality' present in some public reports of the disease and on proposals for screening to establish 'a link between AIDS and homosexuality', which they saw as a campaign to exclude a group of people exercising their rights to 'independence and privacy' (1995:39).

In 1982, the *MMWR* published a set of guidelines in their weekly report on current trends. The report began with the statement that '[t]he etiology of the underlying immune deficiencies seen in AIDS cases is unknown' (1982). Although little was then known about the causes of the disease, it is clear from the overall tone of the report that cases of AIDS were being observed more widely in the USA. This required guidance on the ways in which health care staff should engage with affected individuals while minimising their potential exposure to the disease. In March 1983, the *MMWR* reported that 'since June 1981, over 1200 cases of acquired immune deficiency syndrome (AIDS) have been reported to CDC from 34 states, the District of Columbia, and 15 countries' (1983). The report then described several studies conducted in New York and California and highlighted the existence of a number of different risk behaviours and risk groups. The latter included the 'sexual partners of AIDS patients; sexually active homosexual or bisexual men with multiple partners; Haitian entrants to the United States; present or past abusers of IV drugs; patients with hemophilia' (1983). Confusingly, this particular statement managed not only to conflate risk practices with risk groups, but it also positioned the disease within the context of broader discourses concerning migration to the USA as well as sexuality rights. The report listed a number of groups that had issued statements on prevention, including 'the National Gay Task Force, the National Hemophilia Foundation, the American Red Cross, the American Association of Blood Banks, the Council of Community Blood Centers, the American Association of Physicians for Human

[2] While gay rights activists were successful in de-medicalizing aspects of homosexuality by targeting the prejudices of the medical and public health establishment, they found themselves in a situation where they needed the attention of the same domains if gay men's AIDS-related needs were to be addressed. Given the initial identification of AIDS as a gay disease, there was a clear danger of the re-medicalization of homosexuality. The question then was how to get gay men's health needs addressed without homosexuality being 'remedicalized'.

Rights, and others' (1983). Around the same time, civil society started to become more vocal. Part of the impetus here came from groups concerned with government lack of action on prevention, but part of it arose from growing concern that people with HIV should be treated fairly.

Scientific interest in both this newly identified condition and in emerging cases of AIDS in different places motivated a series of international meetings to consider the situation in the Americas and in Europe in 1983 (Gordenker et al. 1995:37). Parallel to these attempts to deal with the disease, there were already signs from western and central Africa that cases of AIDS were also being identified in some of the countries in the region including Rwanda, Zaire and Zambia. A number of western clinicians made similar observations among African migrant communities in Western Europe (Gordenker et al. 1995:37). One of the first research papers detailing findings from Africa was published in July 1984 by Peter Piot and his colleagues in the *Lancet*. Their paper argued that there was a difference between the epidemiology of AIDS in North America and Western Europe from that of Africa. Writing of their experience in Zaire, they concluded that

> Homosexuality, intravenous drug abuse, and blood transfusion did not appear to be risk factors in these patients. The findings of this study strongly argue that the situation in central Africa represents a new epidemiological setting for this worldwide disease—that of significant transmission in a large heterosexual population. Two instances of clusters of AIDS (not included in the above series) involving males and females with frequent heterosexual contact further implicate heterosexual transmission (Piot et al. 1984: 68).

These were challenging findings as they suggested that the categorization of AIDS as a disease of particular groups was not going to work in framing an international approach. Moreover, their findings also presented a challenge to civil society groups that were trying to get their governments to address their needs in resource-rich settings. In any case, this work led to the first attempts to understand the nature and scale of problem of AIDS within the African region. It is in these attempts that one can see the first steps towards an internationalization of the problem.

One of the first initiatives to try to understand the nature of the disease in non-western contexts was a joint program between the US CDC and Belgian scientists in Zaire who were collaborating with local medical professionals in Kinshasa. It was called Project AIDS and was funded largely by the CDC, the US National Institute of Allergy and Infectious Diseases (NIAID), a part of The US National Institute of Health, with a smaller amount contributed by Belgium's Institute for Tropical Medicine (ITM). The project was led by Jonathan Mann from the US CDC and included Peter Piot among others as scientists who were working in Kinshasa. According to Jon Cohen, the project included more local clinicians than international experts and many of these clinicians were to become leaders in their field in fighting HIV in Africa over the years (Cohen 1997). The project produced many important publications and began to transform ways of thinking about AIDS in resource-poor settings. Due to political changes in Zaire, the project came to an end in 1991 (Cohen 1997).

While the research was innovative it was also limited due to number of ways in which the project approached its work. First, there was only limited involvement by local researchers. As Kakanda Kinjinga, who was interviewed by Cohen and was one of the local scientists on the project said, 'when I was in Project SIDA I didn't even know I was doing research…I really didn't understand the purpose of what we were doing' (1997: 1567). Second, links between the research and the needs of local people with AIDS were weak. According to Bila Kapita, a cardiologist, who was one of the local lead scientists in Zaire, the research needs and public health needs diverged 'I'm sorry to tell you that Projet SIDA had very little impact for infected people here …it would have been useful for them to ask us about what was the useful thing for us they could do here… We knew that AIDS was transmitted by blood transfusion, but nothing was done about it' (1997:1567). Piot himself also acknowledged this tension, 'That's a big discussion we always had: what is the responsibility of what is primarily a research project working with research funds in terms of doing something for the country?' (1997:1567). Third, it was progressively realised that the costs involved in screening blood samples and doing so systematically would be very large indeed and outside the Project's mandate. Finally, differences emerged between CDC and NIAID with respect to the scale and the focus of the overall project (Cohen 1997).

Together, these observations foreground a number of important issues in thinking about the later politics of Global AIDS. First, there is the important leadership role of Jonathan Mann and Peter Piot, among others, which was later to guide the development of a global approach to HIV and AIDS based on the approach described here. Second, there was the relationship between the priorities of the project and local experiences which laid the foundations for later international priority-setting by experts. Third, there was the issue of differences between those most affected in resource-poor settings and those in resource-rich settings, which created a political issue right from the start of international engagement.

Lisk argues that in the period up until 1985, the response to AIDS within the international organizational context was very limited. There are several reasons for this. First, because of the way in which AIDS had been framed, experts 'were not convinced that the disease was a heterosexual problem' (Lisk 2010: 11). Second, AIDS was seen largely as a problem of resource-rich settings where national governments were viewed as being able to deal with problem. Third, there was the legacy of priorities identified in an early WHO meeting convened in 1983 in Denmark, which saw 'safeguarding blood supplies and alerting homosexuals' (2010: 12) as the key issues to be addressed. Here, AIDS was constructed as a infectious disease among gay men, with male homosexuals being designated as the key target group for policy interventions. In both the case of the US CDC and the WHO, organizational mandates and organizational practices influenced their actions and the way in which they approached the issue. The concerns expressed by the WHO, according to Lisk, also linked to the priorities of the CDC, and stressed monitoring and surveillance as well as giving advice on prevention (Gordenker et al. 1995:37). With hindsight, this narrow focus and slow engagement with the disease in resource-poor settings meant that 'WHO missed the initial opportunity to act against the epidemic in Africa and also in the Caribbean' (2010:12).

According to Lisk, WHO and the other international organizations only began to mount a coordinated response to AIDS after 1985 as the result of increasing numbers of AIDS cases. Both his analysis and that provided by and Gordenker et al. highlight the institutional moves that led WHO to lead the international AIDS response, initially in 1986 as a Control Program from within the Division of Communicable Diseases, and then from 1987 as the Global Programme on AIDS (GPA) under Jonathan Mann, who moved to WHO from his CDC role in the Project AIDS in Zaire. In these analyses, the view of the systemic response by international organizations underplays the conditionality of these responses on available knowledge, the ways in which AIDS had initially been categorized as a homosexual disease, and the resistance that was observable at the time in the membership of many other international organizations. For instance, Gordenker et al.'s discussion clearly reveals the tensions underpinning African political engagement with scientific studies demonstrating the existence of AIDS in Africa. Indeed several African countries boycotted 'the first International Symposium on AIDS in Africa convened in Brussels in November 1985' and that those attended 'berated Western media for exaggerating the extent of the epidemic in Africa' (1995:29, also see Cohen 1997). These kinds of reactions presented important political challenges to decision making in the international organizations created and funded by the member states.

Before 1986, scientific efforts to understand what was going on, both in terms of the cause of AIDS and the geographic contexts in which it appeared, internationalized thinking about the disease faster than international organizations themselves could respond, given their formal mandates, membership pressures and vested interests. However, by 1986 several international organizations had caught up with the scientists and the creation of GPA led to a concentrated group of people making headway in developing an international response. This work included getting many countries to create national AIDS plans, building capacity on AIDS across many different contexts, and advising countries in relation to AIDS. At the same time, this work also established WHO as the lead agency in relation to international discussion of the subject. As the lead program on AIDS within the UN system, GPA attracted enormous attention and funding. However, it still remained a sub-unit within WHO. Crucially, GPA was broadly not part of the budgetary structures of the WHO but funded externally. Mann also employed a number of innovative strategies to advance the programme's work. These included the use of a human rights framework to frame discussion, working directly working with non-governmental organizations, and raising AIDS-specific funding. These were challenging approaches for the WHO system. Lisk argues, for instance, that the rights-based approach Mann established raised major questions about infectious disease control more generally. Some argued that 'an approach which excluded screening was not realistic in the context of what was known to be a mass heterosexual epidemic. They evoked the traditional public health approach that calls for action by public authorities to protect society against spread of epidemics' (Lisk 2010:18). On working with local AIDS groups and NGOs, Lisk points out that this was not always easy within the WHO framework at the time, because systems had been built largely to work with medical professionals and health-related segments of national governments (Lisk

2010:19). This in turn presented a challenge to the possibility of operationalizing a rights-based approach to deal with AIDS. Matters became more complicated when GPA needed to coordinate its work with that of other UN bodies such as UNDP, UNICEF and others. This led, for instance, to the creation of a 'UNDP/WHO Alliance to Combat AIDS' (Lisk 2010: 20). Despite the need for collabroation, tension arose when WHO announced its 'Global Commission on AIDS in 1988 to serve as policy guidance for global response' (Lisk 2010: 20).

While WHO clearly wanted to maintain its lead role in the AIDS response, Mann's work in effect created a single-disease response unit that was developing a new approach. And even if WHO was keen on its role as host, it was not easy to shift its work practices and policy-making procedures. This was particularly exacerbated by the fact that by the end of 1980s, GPA was attracting major funding for its work on AIDS and its role started to become better known about than that of WHO itself. A change of leadership at WHO in 1988 made it difficult to maintain this situation. The new Director-General was keen to integrate GPA more fully into WHO management structures. These tensions resulted in the departure of Mann from GPA and a growing dissatisfaction among some donors, which in time led to an external evaluation of its work. The evaluation process highlighted the need for a new interagency approach to the global coordination and leadership of work on AIDS. Importantly, however, it was GPA that established within WHO a more activist approach to engaging with various sectors, and its broadly rights-based outlook as a way of working in this field informed the structure of the new organization that was later to emerge, UNAIDS.

2.2 Meanings of AIDS

In this pre-1996 period, the different dynamics present created a special kind of politics. AIDS had first been identified as a particular disease within a particular community, and different actors, including gay men affected by the disease, policy makers, public health professionals and others found themselves in competition to give meaning to the epidemic. This was important because the framing different actors gave to the epidemic influenced resource allocation to target people's needs. In many cases, the personal experiences of the individuals involved influenced their understanding of AIDS and what it was that the world was now living with. Many key policy actors continued to understand AIDS as a *gay disease*, either from a point of ignorance or based on stigmatizing assumptions about homosexuality and sexually transmitted disease. Others understood the epidemic in different ways. There was a multifaceted process in which both different experiences and varying assumptions about transmission underwrote different ways of thinking about the epidemic. Thus, the politics of AIDS for different actors was about challenging the different meanings of AIDS from different positions (Epstein 1996; Treichler 1999).

From the early 1980s onwards, in North America and in Western Europe people with AIDS had challenged their governments to recognize their citizenship rights to health. A central aspect of this challenge lay in the link mentioned earlier in the CDC report that AIDS overwhelmingly affected gay men. This initial identification of the disease located discussion of the epidemic within the politics of sexuality and with debates about homophobia and conservatism on the one hand, and on the other hand about identity politics and gay rights in resource rich countries. While this clash made AIDS ignorable by the broadly homophobic political establishment, it also provided the grounds on which AIDS community activism to emerge and position AIDS as a health rights problem within the broader context of welfare debates. There were very clear confrontation, for instance, between AIDS activists and the US government throughout the 1980s and the early 1990s, getting the Reagan and G.H.W. Bush governments to rethink their health care provision and drug development and access policies. The political issue here was about the ability of particular group of citizens to exercise their right to demand policy change from government without being marginalized because of their sexuality.

The challenging of public meanings attributed to AIDS was a very important issue for gay men as they had watched many friends die while having access to few public health resources to deal with the circumstances. Their challenge was to show that the political system's stigmatized view of homosexuality was making AIDS as a marginal issue within the broader policy process. To deal with AIDS without prejudice required recognizing and engaging with the community that was experiencing it. For, many policy makers, AIDS did not exist before its identification. However, people living with it thought differently about the situation. Even after its identification, for many policy makers AIDS still did not exist beyond an abstract disease of a sexually *promiscuous* group of people. In the context of policy-making at the time, the dominant meaning of AIDS was informed by the idea of this, rather than by a meaning informed by the experiences of people actually affected by the disease. In this context, policy approaches to the disease and its governance were creating problems. So, the politics of meaning had in this sense very real outcomes for those who were affected by HIV. Activist clashes with government authorities in the US and in western European contexts aimed for forward thinking policy innovations. They sought to fundamentally change the underlying meanings that handicapped the development of appropriate policies (Gould 2009). The meanings in conflict were informed by personal and social experience and in opposition to public policy concerns, and the clashes themselves should be read as attempts to partake in policy process by people who had mostly hitherto been excluded from social policy debate. The politics here was about people with experience of a disease becoming policy actors to challenge the common view of the top-down policy process in which they only appeared as beneficiaries, if they appeared at all. The aim was to bring what it means to live with AIDS to bear on the policy making process rather than policies being made according to a more abstract idea of what AIDS might be.

At around the same time, however, medical experts were tracking the growth of AIDS epidemics in resource-poor settings, particularly in a number of African countries that included Rwanda, Zaire and Zambia. Through their developing world research, they aimed to make AIDS a reality for policy makers so that the epidemic could be dealt with in resource-poor settings. Their goals were, on the one hand, to alert the international development community that this was happening and, on the other hand, to identify the epidemic's mostly heterosexual pattern of transmission as opposed to the pattern seen up to that point in the resource-rich countries. These actions were political from the start as medical scientists had to justify why they needed to study the disease in resource-poor settings and also had to lobby international actors to take their findings seriously. Furthermore, their finding that AIDS in Africa showed a heterosexual pattern of transmission provided an important new challenge in terms of meaning. It prevented the disease from being seen solely an attribute of homosexuals or Haitians. At the same time, it challenged the denial of the existence of the disease in Africa which had based on the initial identification of AIDS as a Western problem affecting gay men. The challenge now was to get the attention of policy makers through different ways of understanding AIDS at a time when there was much reluctance to think about it at all.

In all of these situations, both locally and internationally, people living with AIDS and medical activists articulated their positions on AIDS on the basis of their own experiences. In the case of the first group, people relating their claims to personal experience with AIDS or the experience of it by someone living in the community. In the case of the latter group, medical professionals who were also policy activists used their knowledge based on their clinical experience of people with AIDS in hospitals in resource-poor countries, while also looking at the broader epidemiological data. While these positions allowed for different ways of thinking about AIDS, there was a commonality between them related with the need to convince others of the need for their claims to be recognized and addressed.

In resource-rich contexts, activism was about citizenship rights and calling governments to deliver according to their duty to protect citizens. Particularly with the development of slogans such as *Silence = Death* and the individual targeting of decision makers such as the then President of the USA, Ronald Reagan, activists used a repertoire of tools to engender broader support for their claims (Tilly 2004). In parallel, and on the international front, medical scientists used their expertise and the data they were producing to access to international organizations and to convince policy makers to act. The relatively recent identification of AIDS and its particularities meant that international organizations did not have *know-how* at a basic level. Medical scientists, such as, Jonathan Mann, Peter Piot and others working on AIDS therefore had to be brought in. Without doubt, many international organizations also suffered from homophobia and a reluctance to act on a disease that appeared to impact only a small section of society. In this sense, showing that in resource-poor settings in Africa the pattern of spread was heterosexual was arguably also a strategic deployment of data to influence policy actors. This approach increased the likelihood of a wider range of actors working in international development, such as the World Bank and the UNDP, becoming allies within the international system.

One outcome of these events, which remains a challenge today, derived from a convergence of interest between medical scientists and activists in considering HIV and AIDS from a biomedical perspective. The overarching meaning of the disease was fixed early on when activists asked for immediate medical help. This broadly informed the way policy thinking has continued to understand AIDS. One important reason for this was the fact that medical expertise developed faster than policy thinking and national responses to deal with the disease. However, this framing of the epidemic was not simply the result of medical science, but also linked to the development of treatment activism. This movement particularly in the USA, struggled to get the government to address public health needs by regulating the private pharmaceutical industry's behaviour. Once the meaning of AIDS was fixed as a medical issue, it became the convention. Policy thinking and solutions became linked to the possibility of medical breakthroughs. This situation had practical value for medical scientists. It allowed them to use their expertise to gain access to the international arena. Particularly from 1990 onwards, following US activists' engagement with scientists at the 6th International AIDS Conference in San Francisco, the relationship between activists and scientists was established as a norm. Furthermore, through direct actions such as disrupting scientific and political discussions to challenge prevailing views about AIDS, activists established the procedures that have come to regulate their later engagement with scientists and other civil society groups in the AIDS field (Altman 1994; Patton 1996).

Medical research and the results generated by it was also instrumental in determining the way in which AIDS become part of the international agenda. This happened largely within the established structures and processes of the international health framework. As result, in international fora yet another process of contestation about the meaning of AIDS could be observed. While international organizations approached the disease as a medical problem, their mandates often meant that this meaning had to be adapted according to their operational needs. For instance, for the World Bank and the UNDP AIDS became a health problem that challenged development initiatives, while for the ILO it was a labour issue linked to concerns about health in the work place. In turn, realization of the fact that the disease was becoming commonly observed across international borders signalled the need for policy coordination and led to the establishment of GPA. Furthermore, the realization that the number of people who might have been living with AIDS was potentially much larger than imagined, brought the issue of cost of international policy interventions in resource-poor settings to the fore.

In retrospect, it is clear that many organizations, even some international NGOs, tried to bring AIDS into their work as an 'additional' issue. As a result, coordination of what was being done in relation to AIDS was far from easy. For instance, WHO's mandate allowed it to engage with member states through support and advice to the health sector. The World Bank, and some NGOs funded by this entity as well as by other agencies such as UNDP and UNICEF had a more direct engagement with the field through the implementation of particular programmes. These operational differences were key in influencing how different organizations thought about AIDS as they encountered the disease through their work. They also led to difficulties in the field. Actors involved in community-level action, for example, encountered challenges when AIDS required new thinking about sex and sexuality in resource poor contexts. Some local implementing agencies found themselves facing major political challenges. These included those of a religious, cultural and social nature. AIDS as a medical condition facilitated engagement in diverse contexts as a field of technical expertise. At the same time, the sexual dimensions of AIDS created tensions for some organizations since it required explicit discussion about issues such as on conception, children, the family, pleasure and patriarchal norms. One way of dealing with these challenges was to focus on the narrowly biomedical. But this did not help overcome either the coordination problem created by different mandates at the international level or the many difficulties encountered at the level of policy implementation from stigma and other socio-political constraints.

While international organizations were able to discuss other diseases and, with some reluctance, reproductive health with their member states, the identification of homosexual men as a risk group made it harder for them to consider doing do something about the disease. Homosexuality was considered socially inappropriate at the time and was/is illegal in many countries. As Didier Eribon reminds us, even acknowledging one had HIV in France meant revealing much more than just the information about the disease (2004). This is a relevant way to think more broadly too. On the one hand, mainstream international organizations had to change their thinking and learn how to speak the language of AIDS. On the other hand, they had to have informed discussions with member states to achieve what needed to be achieved. Similarly, more local interventions on AIDS were also facing challenges because AIDS in everyday life signified much more than just a health condition.

These circumstances required more than a simple coordination, as Godenker et al. and Lisk show. Successful coordination required (a) a shared understanding of AIDS, (b) a coordinated policy framework to bring together the different technical, political and financial capacities; (c) the development of common understanding on implementation strategies to engage with different local meanings to influence change, and (d) shared stakes in the outcomes to overcome organizational competition to be seen politically as the most successful organization in dealing with the problem. This was a major challenge in a context where resources were often distributed according to some evident measure of success.

These considerations showed that governance of an issue, in this case AIDS, at the international level required discussion on how to understand and to set priorities for a new problem within the existing structures and organizational practices. This required each organization to go through internal processes of institutionalising AIDS as a part of their overall policy strategies. Then, each organization needed to think about how to coordinate their own work with that of others working on AIDS. And, while individual implementation issues were important to each organization, soon the possibility of creating a coherent, global intervention strategy occupied debate. Given the complexity of the contexts in which AIDS could be observed, a technical approach was needed to bring policy interventions under a coherent framework. The medical approach to AIDS allowed such a coherence to emerge. In the process, however, people with experience of the disease become target groups. This created limits for their political participation, and partaking, in the system.

2.3 Technical Coordination

One of the central issues here was that of creating a shared vision concerning the causes of the disease and those who were most vulnerable to it. While deciding on these might have been challenging, medico-technical descriptions were helpful in arriving at such a shared understanding. They also enhanced the feasibility of policy coordination across different organizational and socio-political settings. As mentioned above, treatment activism and the work of activist medical professionals had already established a pathway. When combined with lack of expertise and urgency, an emergency logic, came to dominate the structuring of Global AIDS. Paraphrasing Stefanos Geroulanos and Todd Meters (2012), one can argue that bit by bit the medical scientific view made life with AIDS comprehensible to the general public in addition to those living with the disease. In this sense, the central technical move lay in defining the disease as a medical problem which created the possibility of there being a shared goal for all actors. This led progressively to the 'institutionalisation' of AIDS as defined by medicine.

This process of grounding coordination to create coherence in a particular scientific understanding of the disease underpinned the framing of Global AIDS. At the same time, however, this approach was about detachment. AIDS is indeed about health and how to sustain health and medicine is an important part of this debate. However, purely medical meanings fail to do justice to the health concerns of particular people living in particular places. Georges Canguilhem's (2012) discussion of the body and health, for example, enables one to see what is being distanced in such a framing of AIDS. He argues that

> ..... the living body is [thus] the singular being whose health expresses the quality of forces that constitute it: it must live with the tasks imposed on it, and it must live exposed to an environment that it does not initially choose. The living body is the totality of the powers of a being that has the capacity to evaluate and represent to itself these powers, their exercise, and their limits...Its health is at once a state and an order (2012:48).

This highlights how AIDS targeted as a global condition detaches itself from AIDS as experienced by particular individuals within the context of their environments. Such a detachment also has political implications since, as discussed earlier, some of initial clashes of meaning were about how to make those people's living with HIV matter for governments to address their needs. The debates underwriting these earlier clashes gradually projected a general understanding of AIDS, in which individuals become subjects of this AIDS lens.

This move, to consider people's lives through an AIDS lens has allowed the development of a general, global approach to the disease. Gradually, the possibility of people's partaking in the global process has become a function of the way in which the global view on AIDS apprehends them. As a result, the politics of Global AIDS emerged as a system of looking at the problems of people through an AIDS lens. This is not based on people's experiences and efforts to make their concerns matter for the public. As a result, arguably, paraphrasing Canguilhem, AIDS became a disease 'that is publicized' and, in this, the patient has become dependent on this way of being made public (2012: 49).

Another aspect of this move towards global coherence and coordination was related to the growing push by donors (witnessed through the 1990s) to understand how the money on AIDS was spent. While this was an important step, it followed what Gordenker et al. see as a path dependency within organizations (1995:42). In most cases, as Baldwin (2005) argues, existing ways of acting on infectious disease informed how organizations reacted to AIDS (Baldwin 2005). For instance, given WHO's mandate for assisting developing countries on health matters, HIV debate in resource rich settings at the time created a situation whereby WHO considered the initial emergence of AIDS as being outside its mandate. The challenge derived from the fact that on the one hand there existed a model for fighting infectious disease that sought to act immediately, while on the other hand dealing effectively with AIDS required engaging with local sensitivities about sex, sexuality and sexually transmitted disease. Moreover, while an emergency response facilitated action, it ignored the different meanings carried by AIDS and how people lived with it in different parts of the world.

GPA was certainly key in the creation of a global view using the technical approaches to international coordination developed from within WHO. By making Global AIDS the main target for policy thinking, GPA was able to demonstrate how a coordinated international agenda could be made compatible with organizational mandates. This technical approach also helped think about ways of both keeping AIDS as a priority over time and generating enough resources – in the form of funding – to deal with the situation in resource-poor settings. Here, the funding concerns and coordinating funding for the GPA and its policy initiatives became an important aspect of the politics of AIDS within the international system. As Lisk (2010) highlights, the funding that the GPA attracted created its own set of problems as it was within the WHO structure while receiving targeted funds independent of the WHO (2010). The potential for a serious deterioration of circumstances in Africa in particular, with millions of people dying, provided legitimacy to this approach for internationally coordinated action and for the funding for it.

Jonathan Mann's approach in GPA was also instrumental in developing new work practices as part of international AIDS work. Considering the lack of AIDS expertise within many organizations, Mann considered working with civil society groups was important, in that they had more expertise at that stage. He therefore encouraged GPA to work closely with these groups. This approach resonated with some UN organizations such as the World Bank, while for others it posed a challenge as they considered themselves the exclusive supporters of state-oriented activities. Furthermore, civil society actors brought into this environment first-hand experiences and the challenges of dealing with AIDS in resource-poor settings. For civil society groups, this move towards inclusion enabled them to deploy their activism within the international arena in challenging governments to deal with AIDS. In this way, the moral challenge created by conditions in resource-poor settings became a moral challenge at the international level and a call on authorities to act to stop people dying. Arguably, it is through these connections to AIDS activism and the use of a citizens' rights approach, that Mann tried to construct a rights-based agenda for international policy to deal with the disease. This attempt to respond to AIDS using a rights-based approach differed from an emergency approach to infectious disease control and presented a major political challenge to governments in many countries.

Together, these debates highlight the dynamics of the politics of AIDS within the international context with different motivations driving different actors' behaviour, the way they thought about AIDS and inter-agency competition to access to resources. The reluctance of many governments to engage with these debates also motivated international actors to think about the need to have a coherent global approach. This required constructing a global meaning for the disease that would underwrite coordination.

2.4 Conclusion

In this chapter, the critical issue has been to understand the way in which competing ways of thinking on AIDS informed the development of a common understanding on AIDS as a global issue. The views that went into this mix came from different locations ranging from people with first hand experiences of the disease, to local activists, to health professionals to national and international policy makers. Activist engagement with policy makers in the USA and the other resource-rich countries over time changed various governments' understanding and approach to the disease. These engagements and their outcomes were also internationalized in the sense that activists' networks information and learning were shared across resource rich settings and in many contexts government behaviour was influenced by them overtime. A major focus of political debate, to stress it once again, was about the need for gay men to have recognition, to partake as equal citizens and to have their needs addressed as citizens. This relationship, once internationalized, presented a challenge both for activists and their own governments to engage with anything outside their own context. Furthermore, given the conservative and often homophobic nature of government responses across the spectrum, these governments were unlikely to engage in any meaningful discussion within international organizations about this disease and its implications in resource-poor settings.

The overall international political context was defined by struggles within a citizenship rights framework and the possibility of internationalizing the outcomes of these struggles to address the needs of people in resource-poor settings. This of course required having a sufficiently general view of the problem, AIDS, for this step to be taken. It is within this context that Jonathan Mann and others tried to internationalize concern about the situation in the resource-poor settings and, more importantly, do something about it. Here, it is important to emphasize that Mann and others were trying to voice the needs of those people who were fighting AIDS in their lives. The struggles that took place throughout the late 1980s and the early 1990s were as much about creating incentives for resource rich countries to engage with the disease in developing countries, as they were about paying attention to what was happening closer to home. The idea of Global AIDS as a coherent framing to motivate policy thinking emerged at the juncture of these experiences and motivations to deal with the disease. It was centrally structured, as described above, by a medical and emergency approach. In time, the possibility of dealing with AIDS became framed with the Global AIDS lens. Gradually, people's lives, as suggested by Canguilhem, thereby became considered at 'the discretion of' the social relations underwriting this lens (2012: 49).

Chapter 3
The Institutionalization of Global AIDS and the Creation of the Joint United Nations Programme on HIV/AIDS (UNAIDS)

In the previous chapter, I analyzed the context within which the idea of stronger coordination for a coherent international AIDS response emerged. In that process I observe emerging lines of sometimes competing arguments and contours of thinking about HIV as a global disease. Building on this, the focus of this chapter is on the creation of the Joint United Nations Programme on HIV/AIDS (UNAIDS) and how this new formation institutionalized a global AIDS perspective. The demands recognized as part of this creation included the need for a coherent and shared understanding of AIDS; coherent and robust data on the disease and on infection rates; coordinated policy frameworks to bring the technical and political capacities of international organizations together for coherent policy intervention in multiple country contexts; a shared understanding of expected outcomes; and a reliable source of financial support for international programming and intervention.

Prior to the creation of UNAIDS, numerous international organizations had dealt with the epidemic in manner linked to their internal decision making processes and policy practices (Gordenker et al. 1995: 42 and Baldwin 2005). The creation of UNAIDS marked a shift in the way the international system attempted to engage with AIDS as a policy concern. Considering the objectives set for the organization, which will be described below, the new institution was also tasked with developing a global understanding of the disease and, in turn, with sharing this understanding. The creation of the UNAIDS and the development of its approach to AIDS is perhaps best viewed as an institutional process leading to a 'conceptual system' that has framed how AIDS came to be understood globally (Descombes 2014: 301). This was achieved through the policy development and public communication practices of the new organization, which together constituted the global meanings of AIDS and created through this a powerful impetus for political action. As Descombes has argued, 'common meanings bring together [...] partners who must do different things and whose roles and statuses are determined by an established rule, a social custom that they both follow' (2014: 301). Seen in this way, UNAIDS was in fact tasked by creating the social customs and established rules to guide its cosponsors' policy work in this field as well as broader policy interventions by other actors,

H. Seckinelgin, *The Politics of Global AIDS*, Social Aspects of HIV 3,
DOI 10.1007/978-3-319-46013-0_3

including national governments and civil society groups. In time, this work to create and support the use of such a common set of understandings of the disease gave rise to the politics of Global AIDS.

UNAIDS did this through – among other activities – advocacy and the circulation of policy guidelines which succeeded in diffusing its approach throughout a range of international and national policy contexts (Hacking 1995; Descombes 2014). This process both created and maintained the way in which Global AIDS was generally understood. It also positioned AIDS in a particular way within international politics with such force that whenever AIDS or its politics are considered today, we encounter these ideas within the context created by UNAIDS' initial framing of the issues. It is therefore important to unpack this process of institutionalization of meaning and its reproduction with UNAIDS at its centre. In doing so, it is important to recognise that what we encounter as Global AIDS is the outcome of the way in which AIDS has been developed into a coherent policy issue through competition, contestation, negotiation and cooperation. From the perspective of politics as taking-part in a process with others to influence different publics, UNAIDS itself can be seen as the outcome of the politics of AIDS at multiple levels during this period. The structure of the organization also reflects these political contestations. At the time of its creation, and in the early years at least, UNAIDS provided an important space for politics as taking-part. Through its many policy initiatives, UNAIDS influenced other actors' behaviour in many different ways,[1] most usually using 'three symbolic elements' to position itself and frame AIDS as a global problem, through 'problem ownership (… who claims a say in defining a problem); causality (… which theory of causes and consequences of the situation is publically espoused?) and accountability (… who is praised and blamed for [failing to] solve the problem)' (Gusfield 1981: 6–7).

In this chapter, I want to consider two of these three elements and the way in which they became instrumental in reproducing a particular view on AIDS. In particular, I want to focus on the way in which the formation of UNAIDS enabled the organization to have the authority to define the problem, and how in the process the internal structuring of the organization moved towards a global AIDS solidarity which underpins the accountability of the system. I will consider the third element – causality – in a later chapters.

3.1 Forming UNAIDS

The name of the new organizational formation in itself signified a very different approach. UNAIDS was conceived as an organization with responsibility for coordinating UN-wide HIV policy initiatives. Because of this, it involved contributions from all the participating organizations both on know-how in particular issue areas and also in the form of the joint funding of its structures. The creation of UNAIDS

[1] In a sense UNAIDS is one of the 'globalizers' described by Ngirae Woods (2006).

was also underwritten by experience that simply having a common interest will not by itself allow different organizations to coordinate their work. Furthermore, an apparent common interest on an issue, in this case AIDS, does not necessarily create a community with a common understanding and approach. UNAIDS in this way represented a new way of thinking about organizational development within the UN system to deal with cross-cutting issues.

The creation of UNAIDS was endorsed by the Economic and Social Council of the UN (ECOSOC) resolutions 1994/24 and E/1995 L.24/Rev.1. Resolution 1994/24 was passed at the 44th plenary meeting of the Council on 26 July 1994 after the noting of various debates, consultations and decisions within a number of UN related organizations including the World Bank 'to undertake a joint and a co-sponsored United Nations Programme on HIV/AIDS, on the basis of co-ownership, collaborative planning and execution and equitable sharing of responsibility'. The resolution stated that

> [E]mphasizing that the global HIV/AIDS epidemic affects every country of the world and its magnitude and impact are greatest in developing countries, [E]mphasizing also the urgent need to mobilize all United Nations system organizations and other development partners in the global response to HIV/AIDS, in coordinated manner and according to the comparative advantage of each organization, [ECOSOC] endorses the establishment of a joint and co-sponsored United Nations programme on HIV/AIDS (1994: 1).

In many ways, this is an interesting statement in itself as it says explicitly that UNAIDS was to be a programme and not a new organization. Furthermore, collaborative work at all levels was considered to be its main means of functioning.[2] ECOSOC's endorsement of this new approach was justified by the unprecedented growth of the epidemic across many countries.

An understanding of the global nature of AIDS is also implicit in these statements. The global here is linked to the appearance of the disease in multiple country contexts and connected to the UN's mandate of engaging with member states that need help in dealing with the disease. The ECOSOC resolution set January 1996 as the moment at which the new programme should begin. After requesting six sponsoring agencies to find a director and other staff, ECOSOC urged 'the six-sponsors, through the committee to initiate as soon as possible programme activities at the country level', and stressed that

> priority should be given to programme's activities at the country level, where the response to the urgent needs and problems posed by HIV/AIDS should be focused, and underlines the importance of the programme's country level operations' functioning within the framework of national plans and priorities and a strengthened resident coordinator system (1994: 1).

These stipulations reveal something of a debate between donor agencies working in developing countries and other policy actors. Donor agencies demanded a more

[2] Another way of thinking about this might be to consider UNAIDS creation as an attempt to create a formal 'policy network that would 'create *de facto* linkages between those controlling formal governance arrangements and those engaged in the sub-politics of running the normal, day to day or socio-technical practices in less formal …arrangements on the ground' (Hoppe 2011: 121).

coordinated and systematic approach to HIV-related intervention to deal with rapidly expanding programmes in resource-poor settings. Here, we can see an early indication of an issue that would later become more central politically, as well as the underlying motivation to discuss AIDS as a global problem. The establishment of UNAIDS was about how to balance the need for coordination with country-level interventions that were trying to address particular needs. This was not a simple balancing act. It involved translating country-level needs into the priorities of international actors and their donors. The role that UNAIDS played in this task was to establish a global understanding of AIDS within the international policy context. Before analysing this further, I want though to look at the structure of the new programme as it was set out in response to the ECOSOC resolution of 1994 and then in the Memorandum of Understanding on UNAIDS signed by its co-sponsors.

3.2 The Organizational Structure of UNAIDS

The new programme was initially co-sponsored by the United Nations Development Programme (UNDP), the United Nations Children's Fund (UNICEF), the United Nations Fund for Population Activities (UNFPA), the United Nations Educational, Scientific and Cultural Organization (UNICEF), the World Health Organization (WHO) and the World Bank. The ECOSOC resolution set out the objectives of the new programme under 6 sub-paragraphs. The first objective described the general direction of travel. It stated that the programme was to 'provide global leadership in response to the epidemic' (1994: 3). It made it clear that the new programme would have to go beyond simply coordinating AIDS work within the UN system. UNAIDS would need to *lead* the global response by producing a particular kind of knowledge and by engaging with different actors. This acknowledged implicitly the importance of the expertise on HIV that had already emerged through GPA as a precursor to UNAIDS, as well as the importance of building on that expertise within the new programme. It also highlighted the lack of such expertise in many other organizations including the co-sponsors. The second and third objectives set out the reach of the programme to 'achieve and promote global consensus on policy and programmatic approaches' (1994: 3), and the importance of developing these policy and programmatic approaches. These established a wide and deep reach for the programme considering the emphasis put on country-level engagement by ECOSOC. This view was further strengthened by the 4th objective that explicitly tasked the programme with engaging with national governments. A 5th objective allowed the new programme to be flexible in the way it engaged with diverse actors whom could act within the epidemic, as it is required UNAIDS to 'promote broad-based political and social mobilization to prevent and respond to HIV/AIDS within countries, ensuring that national responses involve a wide range of sectors and institutions' (1994: 3). This is particularly significant as it built on GPA's experience, which had included civil society and community organizations in its work. This objective took matters further however by making the inclusion of these groups an organizational imperative. Arguably, it also highlighted the way in which negotiations surrounding the establishment of UNAIDS were influenced by civil society activists, both within the UN system and beyond. Finally, the new programme was also recognized as an advocate for political leadership at all of the levels it is supposed to work at, which included resource allocation and funding.

This short list of objectives supported by section IV of the resolution provided the structural orientation for the new programme. The objectives set out its role in political and technical terms, which include monitoring trends and knowledge creation to develop programmatic interventions. The new programme was to be politically involved in a wide range of areas – from leadership to advocacy for particular programmes – while at the same time being tasked to develop ways of thinking on policies to deal with HIV. The link between leadership and policy development objectives was considered through its tasking to get things done at a local level, as well as by creating policy consensus within the international system. In this attempt to build an institutionalized coherence to deal with the challenges posed by AIDS, the objectives established the programme as politically responsible for the creation of common framework for thinking about and responding to AIDS as an international policy issue. The ultimate aim therefore was to 'solve' the AIDS problem. According to Hoppe (2011: 101), this was in many ways a 'world-making' process that involved creating a view on AIDS that informed the rationality of all actors in tackling the defined problem.

At the same time, however, there was also the challenge that had been recognized by Descombes as the 'logical problem of the representation of action whose agent is in the plural' (2014: 126). The plurality of the agency here was linked to the fact that UNAIDS was a joint programme and relied on the resources of its different cosponsors. The political agency of UNAIDS, formed in line with ECOSOC objectives, needed to be balanced with the exercise of that agency in collaboration with others. The tensions associated with this were observed by Franklyn Lisk. He points out that in parallel budgetary debates surrounding UNAIDS 'some donors wanted to fund only a small Secretariat with only policy and program coordination functions' (2010: 34). This is an interesting observation as the objectives set out by the original ECOSOC resolution were much more ambitious. The point of contention here was that some sponsors thought that 'the bulk of the new program's money should go directly to the co-sponsoring agencies to support their own HIV/AIDS activities' (Lisk 2010: 34). Discussion on funding at this stage can therefore be seen as a tactical way in which some sponsors' sought to control the political agency attributed to UNAIDS. This involved questioning the overall mandate created for UNAIDS independent of the work done by individual cosponsors in this field.

While the ECOSOC resolution outlined the objectives of the new programme with clarity, work on the structuring and functions of the new organization was not finalized by the resolution. In its preamble, under point 4, the resolution calls on sponsoring organizations to 'transform inter-agency working group into a formally constituted Committee of Co-sponsoring Organizations (CCO). This was supposed to comprise of 'the heads of those organizations, or their specifically designated representatives, which would function in a rotational chairmanship, establish a transition team and assume interim responsibility …overseeing the transition process leading to the full implementation of the programme' (1994). The CCO effectively became the forum through which the staff of the new programme were to be appointed and its budget to be decided upon. It was also tasked to develop 'the composition of the programme coordinating board (PCB)' as the main governance forum for the programme once it was launched. Taking decisions on the PCB's composition had important implications for the overall outcomes of the UNAIDS' work. The CCO recognized the importance of appointing a director for the new programme and wanted that person to join the committee in its transition work to ensure leadership of the new programme. The CCO proposed that Peter Piot be appointed to the secretary general of the UN in December 1995. Piot was well-known both from his work with GPA and as a leading scientist in the AIDS field. Once he had been appointed, and from 1995 onwards, under his leadership the CCO began to shape the structures and direction of the new programme (Lisk 2010: 26–36). These debates and the appointment of Piot stimulated a step change in ongoing discussions on the role of WHO in relation to the epidemic. His appointment enabled the new programme to learn from GPA experience while also locating medical expertise at the top of the new programme. This would enable the programme to use this expertise both to comparative advantage with co-sponsors and as political leverage in policy debates.

It was clear from the beginning that Piot approached the objectives set by the ECOSOC resolution in their widest possible interpretation. He took political agency very seriously. His goal was to create not only a coherent global AIDS policy framework but also a global community committed to and working on HIV. As Lisk points out, Piot lobbied for a kind of PCB that reflected the spirit of the ECOSOC objectives and included members from outside the sponsoring organization or governments. This was linked with his experience in GPA of developing relationships with non-governmental actors. However, considering the centrality of the PCB to the new programme, a number of cosponsors were not keen on the idea of including non-state actors in decision-making processes. In the end, the compromise was to include NGO representatives in the PCB but as non-voting members. This highlighted different ways of thinking about what would work when engaging with HIV globally. While a conventional approach might prioritise states, the position based on the experience of Piot and colleagues in the field suggested that civil society and networks of civil society organizations ought also to be part of the intervention strategies. Using that experience to negotiate seems to have produced the compromise. The outcome of non-voting membership was to impact on NGO contributions in the long-term, but it was an unprecedented move to include them in decision-making at organizational level within the UN system (Seckinelgin 2009a). It also indicated symbolically that the new programme was committing itself directly to those living with the disease. These key moves in the formation of UNAIDS created a collective and a 'community' around AIDS, or at least more of a collective than was usually expected of an international organization. At the same time, they helped create a common understanding of AIDS as a global issue. The idea was ripe to establish a community of actors – an 'us all' – that had a shared stake in the global AIDS arena.

By the time that UNAIDS was launched in January 1996, it had a much larger secretariat than the CCO was initially keen on (Lisk 2010). Piot used the ECOSOC objectives to create a programme, which in a very short period of time after 1996, acquired the outlook of an international organization. This was a major development given that the link with WHO in terms of UNAIDS finances remained very close (through the UNAIDS Trust created by the WHO to fund the new programme's operations). For many, UNAIDS was seen as a specialized agency within the UN, with most people not understanding the description of it as a Joint Programme. UNAIDS approach to building community required a tactical approach facilitating the new programme's relationship with governments in the field. This allowed UNAIDS to project more of an activist and solidarity-based identity while still being an international organization. Gradually, it projected an image of an organization that brought people living with HIV, and knowledge based on their experiences, closer to and into the international system.

3.3 Institutionalization of the Global Lens

The memorandum of understanding signed by the co-sponsoring organizations aligned with the objectives set by the ECOSOC and also reiterated commitment to co-funding the organization. It is interesting to note that other UN system organizations later signed the memorandum to become sponsors, including the United Nations Drug Control Programme in 1999 and the International Labour Organization in 2001. In its section 3 of the memorandum, which focuses on Cosponsorship, paragraph 3.1 highlights the technical relationship as follows

> UNAIDS will draw upon the experience and strengths of [the] Cosponsoring Organization to develop its HIV/AIDS-related polices, strategies and technical guidelines, which will be incorporated by each of them into their policy strategy mainstream, subject to their governance processes and reflected in the activities of their own mandate.

It is then stated that 'the activities of the Cosponsoring Organizations relating primarily to HIV/AIDS at global level shall be within the context of the global work plan of UNAIDS, developed in collaboration with the Cosponsoring Organizations' (1995: 2). In these paragraphs, the technical expertise of UNAIDS is recognized as the guiding force in relation to the epidemic. Once again the leading role of UNAIDS is recognized while being underwritten by the cosponsors. In the end, the centrality of the UNAIDS Secretariat in developing global policies, intervention and implementation strategies on behalf of the totality of the cosponsors, albeit with their support, was set.

In the language of some international organizations, a level of concern can be observed at this stage. Several of them, including WHO, the World Bank[3] and UNICEF wanted to control how they engaged with HIV and AIDS from within their own mandate. A second step towards framing UNAIDS as the lead coordinating agency lies in the Section VIII of the memorandum on the Global Level. Paragraph 8.1 states that 'at [the] global level, UNAIDS will provide support in policy formulation, strategic planning, technical guidance, research and development, advocacy and external relations'. The document then goes on to say that

> Working closely with the appropriate organizations, UNAIDS will also support normative activities relating to HIV/AIDS in areas such as social and economic planning, population, culture, education, health, community, development and social mobilization, sexual and reproductive health, and women and adolescents (1995: 5).

Through this step, a central political position is carved out for UNAIDS within the international policy context to frame normative debate on HIV for collective use.

In statements such as these, the memorandum of understanding established the way in which UNAIDS would come to govern cosponsorship. Furthermore, the knowledge and expertise deficit within the international system more generally placed UNAIDS in a governing position. UNAIDS mandate allowed the organization to present itself as being 'in control of the problematic situation, that is, in a position and endowed with resources to remedy it' (Hoppe 2011: 102), which in turn led to a situation where the organization knew 'how to specify what the solution to the problem looks like' (Hoppe 2011: 102). The memorandum provides some acceptance of this role by the other actors, including the civil society groups involved.

With this rethinking came an organizational challenge: namely, how far was this organizational mandate compatible with wider global AIDS horizons? Within a very short period of time, efforts were made to mainstream the AIDS lens developed and maintained by UNAIDS into other sectors. In order to participate with legitimacy in international AIDS work, actors had to look at their work through this lens. UNAIDS ability to achieve such an outcome derived from its role in establishing norms about the way in which to do HIV-related work. The memorandum of understanding not only allowed UNAIDS to develop its leadership role on AIDS but also legitimated the process of establishing a comprehensive discourse on HIV and AIDS that underwrote the global view. In particular, paragraph 8.1 of the memorandum, discussed earlier, allowed this step to be taken by UNAIDS. Furthermore, through the inclusion of civil society groups, the joint and co-sponsored organization became the centre of a community of solidarity. What ultimately made UNAIDS's approach so successful was that it posited 'multiplicity as a unity' in the face of a major problem (Descombes 2014: 132).

[3] Arguably, this can be also observed in the fact that the World Bank signed the Memorandum of Understanding in 1996.

Given the nature of AIDS activism, which I will discuss later, this was also a strategic choice which allowed the UNAIDS to differentiate itself from other organisations, through the authority gained by being closer to people with HIV than others. By tactically combining being close to civil society with having concentrated medical expertise, UNAIDS developed its own view on the kind of knowledge-base that was most relevant for global policy interventions.

3.4 External Dynamics

Without doubt, the establishment of a specialized UN programme focusing on one disease highlights the urgency of global policy development. UNAIDS, by providing an explanation for this new approach to disease control, focused the public's attention by framing AIDS as a global emergency. The aim here organizationally was both to justify its funding needs[4] and to show its added value to the larger community in solving the global AIDS problem. The challenge was, and has been, to represent AIDS as a problem that requires unified action by the international system and to keep the focus on it. There were a number of important challenges in doing so.

Firstly, the debate within resource rich settings was about citizens and their right to health within a bounded community. The problem and its solution were based on citizens' rights claims whose terms were difficult to translate into an international context. It is not a simple policy matter to make millions of people's situation an issue and keep it at the centre of the international political agenda. UNAIDS' ability to project itself as an organization of solidarity and community, was instrumental in dealing with these challenges. Concern for the state of AIDS globally had to be projected internationally to facilitate its role of influencing other organizations, including its cosponsors, both to understand the global nature of the problem and what needed to be done within a global policy framework. One key way of doing this was to frame the problem as an emergency. In this way, UNAIDS created a humanitarian imperative and became a voice for AIDS community in challenging broader publics. This practice of projecting both AIDS globally as an emergency and the need for unified response, also allowed UNAIDS to create an understanding of the disease, messaged strongly as 'we are all part of the response'.

Secondly, the politics of creating a global community was also affected by the drive to display solidarity with people with HIV in resource poor settings. The possibility of resource rich governments dealing both with AIDS-related needs in their countries and also helping people in resource-poor settings raised concerns about resource allocation. As UNAIDS began its work, effective antiretroviral therapy was

[4] UNAIDS' core budget for 1998–1999 period was 89.4 million USD, provided as contributions from governments, cosponsors and income enlisted as other income (UNAIDS 1999a PCB(8)). Reading earlier budget statements clearly revealed that the objectives set for the UNAIDS were more ambitious than the budget it had received.

becoming a possibility in resource rich settings. In these contexts, this was a game-changer as many people were able to access medications that worked and rethink their lives in a different way. This change had a number of important implications: (a) confrontational activism in these contexts gradually disappeared and civil society responses to AIDS became more professionalized; (b) governments become more responsive to HIV as there was now a medical way to address activists' demands; and (c) activists considered how best they could utilize their expertise towards other ends.

These developments carried various implications for international debate and for UNAIDS in particular. This change allowed for a repositioning global AIDS debate towards resource-poor settings without creating competition either for attention or immediate resources. It allowed UNAIDS to focus its work on poorer countries and bring the needs of marginalised communities to the centre of international debate. It also enabled activists from resource rich settings, who had gained enormous political and policy experience, to put their expertise to work in the international policy context within the newly created UNAIDS. These crossovers brought new experiences and models of policy activism into UNAIDS as well as into the growing international NGO community that was focused on HIV and AIDS.

In order to maintain leadership of this approach UNAIDS developed new practices in data collection, monitoring, evaluation and reporting, alongside new intervention strategies to fulfil this role. These processes aimed to produce the knowledge and policy frameworks that built on understanding AIDS as a global problem. They translated 'global AIDS insights into control, constraint and leverage factors into detailed, custom-made action plans' for different actors participating in this collective work (Hoppe 2011: 102). It soon became clear that UNAIDS had become both a political actor and a space for politics. In order to be able to participate in this space, however, actors needed to negotiate how they would contribute to the global AIDS horizons set by UNAIDS. And by participating in these processes, other organizations including individual governments, civil society groups and people who were living with HIV, become part of the wider global AIDS community. Through their inclusion, they also created through their own activities the space within which UNAIDS exercised its competence in monitoring, evaluating and guiding AIDS polices. Therefore, it is perhaps not surprising that UNAIDS gradually came to frame the global politics of AIDS through its own practices, through what it did to assess the state of AIDS, and through what it presented as being the best response to the disease.[5]

[5] The content and expanding size of the annual state of the AIDS reports, which are usually released on 1st December as part of international AIDS Day activities, provide good examples in this.

3.5 UNAIDS Reports as a Practice of Institutionalization

In one of the earliest reports from UNAIDS entitled the *Report on the Global HIV/AIDS Epidemic – June 1998*, we can get a glimpse of some of these issues and the way in which UNAIDS was trying to deal with them. The report begins by framing the scale of the problem. In its presentation of this, both visual materials and narrative are used to highlight different burdens of the disease in different parts of the world, set out in broad terms. By presenting the visual material in conjunction with the basic numbers of 30 million people living with HIV/AIDS and their distribution across the globe, the document makes it immediately clear where the resource-poor countries were and, in particular, that AIDS in Africa was a major problem.

Beyond this, the style of presentation – much used since – immediately establishes the global nature of the disease and enables global comparisons to be made visually using a map of the globe. The narrative of the report builds on this imagery to show the imbalanced disease burden in developing countries and the implications of this situation for those living with HIV. The tone of the introductory pages is sombre. It is stated that the trajectory of the situation is likely to get worse and that many more lives will be lost: 'these deaths will not be the last; there is worse to come. The virus continues to spread causing nearly 16 000 infections a day' (1998: 7). This statement also places a humanitarian response to this emergency situation on the agenda. The narrative is constructed in compelling way, with AIDS being discussed as a global problem that involves everyone.

> Today, although one in every 100 adults in the most sexually active age bracket (15–49) is living with HIV, only a tiny fraction know about their infection. Because people can live for many years with HIV before showing any sign of illness, the virus can spread unobserved for a long time. In the face of other pressing concerns, it has been relatively easy in many parts of the world for political, religious and community leaders to overlook the significance of the epidemic. But AIDS cases, and AIDS deaths, are growing the world over, and there are few countries where it is still possible to be ignorant of the scale of the disease. Some 2.3 million people died of AIDS during the course of 1997…Indeed HIV/AIDS is among the top ten killers worldwide, and given current levels of HIV infection, it may soon move into the top five, overtaking such well-established causes of death as diarrhoeal diseases (1998: 7).

This extract provides a good example of the disease-centric narrative that was to dominate the UNAIDS response. In it, people living with HIV and the specific conditions under which they experience the disease are subsumed within the global gaze of the international organization. The point of this is to show that the disease is everywhere. The representation uses numbers to show the size of the disease burden to create affect, but also the global stakes in thinking properly and carefully about HIV disease. In other words, this is a narrative that was constructed as a tool to facilitate the development of UNAIDS' global mandate and to create political momentum for unified action.

Another aspect of this mode of presentation can be seen in a paragraph on mother-to-child infection (1998: 8). The infection rates presented set out the case dramatically by showing that already 2.7 million children under 15 had died by 1997. This is discussed in general terms without talking about the specific distribution of the experience of disease among children (1998: 8). Once this image of a global stake in the problem has been created, the report then turns to resource-poor countries, where it is said

> As the fold-out map at the end of this report shows, HIV infections are concentrated in the developing world, mostly in countries least able to afford to care for infected people. In fact, 89 % of people with HIV live in sub-Saharan Africa and the developing countries of Asia, which between them account for less than 10 % of global Gross National Product (1998: 8).

This paragraph serves to transition the effect by looking at the situation in different regions and different categories of people living with the disease. The report continues

> from the beginning of the epidemic until the start of 1998, some 8.2 million children around the world had lost their mother to AIDS. Many of those had lost their fathers as well. In 1997 alone, around 1.6 million children were orphaned by HIV; over 90 % of those orphans live in sub-Saharan Africa (1998: 9).

The narrative that follows makes it clear that many millions more have been infected in Africa than anywhere else, with serious and dramatic consequences. In its consideration of each region, the report points to s different patterns of infection. For instance, it talks about Africa as experiencing a more generalized epidemic, while in Latin America HIV transmission has been greatest among communities such as men who have sex with men. In Eastern Europe, people who inject drugs are among those most affected.

The overall image presented by this report is one that seeks to show the scale and depth of the problem. It also offers a certain mapping of the HIV epidemic. Each issue is discussed in reference to a number of countries with the report providing information about how different countries are dealing with the epidemic and where infection rates are increasing. Not much space is given to an analysis of the causes in particular situations. The primary aim is to offer a global view.

Another important feature of the report lies in what it has to say about the industrialized world. Here, it points to a decline in infection and mortality rates. Although the report acknowledges the importance of safer sex prevention measures, it argues that this decrease is primarily due to newly available drug treatment in these areas (1998: 18). The possibility of treatment access is presented as a more remote possibility in developing countries:

> In industrialized nations, a few countries in Latin America, and Thailand, many people who test positive for HIV have access to combination antiretroviral therapy which reduces the amount of HIV in the body and delays the onset of AIDS. In other countries combination antiretroviral therapy is also used, but by a very small proportion of HIV-infected people. Such therapies are expensive, hard to administer, and require regular medical monitoring (1998: 46).

The reasons listed here mostly relate to economic, distributive and policy issues rather than to the environmental constraints within which people in most developing countries live. This narrative suggests that while UNAIDS attempts to offer a global view on AIDS, this view is limited to what it was thought reasonable to do at that stage of the epidemic, given available knowledge and resources. In other words, its expert knowledge underwrites the way in which AIDS should be understood as a global issue independent of the needs of particular contexts.

The report is also notable for its methodological concerns. The development of a global perspective requires specific methods to be deployed to assess the state of the disease. There is a clear emphasis on how to improve information flows globally and how best to establish baseline measurements in developing countries. It is also clear that more accurate and detailed information is available from industrialized countries compared to developing countries. The methods approaches promoted by UNAIDS are presented and their relevance to global monitoring and policy support discussed. These are important delineations because they establish the expertise of a relatively new organization and underwrite the relevance of its global knowledge production for policy intervention.

The UNAIDS report that followed in 1999 was presented in a different way. While it still contains a global mapping of the disease and highlights emerging issues within that context, it also showcases UNAIDS as a new entity and discusses why its work is so important. This is done up front in a Preface by the Executive Director, Peter Piot. The first sentence of this is worth looking at because it encapsulates the position that would come to symbolise UNAIDS outlook in later years. Piot begins by stating that:

> We live at a turning point in human history. AIDS spotlights all that is strong and weak in humanity: our vulnerability and fears, as well as our strength and compassion, especially for those more vulnerable, less able, or poorer than ourselves (1999b: 7).

This prophetic tone, which is used many times in later UNAIDS reports, is a key feature which enabled AIDS to be kept on the international agenda. The language here is 'world-making' in the sense of asserting the emergence of a Global AIDS 'groupthink' (Hoppe 2011: 110). In the lines that follow, the state of AIDS across the world is described,

> These deaths will not be the last – there is worse to come. Every year AIDS takes new directions: India and South Africa, both relatively untouched only a few years ago, now have among the fastest-growing epidemics in the world. New AIDS epidemics are emerging with frightening speed in Eastern and Central Europe. And sub-Saharan Africa remains the hardest-hit region in the world. Globally, young people –those who must build the bridges, create national wealth and conduct the research of the future – experience half of all new HIV infections. In many parts of the world, AIDS is the single greatest threat to economic, social and human development (UNAIDS 1999b: 7).

While the data underwriting this statement were available at the time of the 1998 report, the tone of this statement frames the situation in terms of a major global disaster. The first line above is almost a threat intended to force policy makers to pay attention. Piot then moves on to describe the role of UNAIDS in the process to fight AIDS:

> In the face of these enormous and frightening challenges, the strength to fight back comes from pooling our resources and working together. Founded just three years ago, in 1996,

> UNAIDS is an innovative joint programme that brings together the expertise and efforts of its seven Cosponsors – UNICEF, UNDP, UNFPA, UNDCP, UNESCO, WHO, the World Bank. Each of them has increased action against HIV/AIDS in its own sphere and is actively contributing to the UNAIDS response (1999b: 7).

This positioning highlights the importance of UNAIDS and its centrality to the response. Although the co-sponsoring agencies are mentioned, it is clear that it is the UNAIDS Secretariat's own work that will be leading the effort in this area. Piot then lists some of the successes already achieved in creating leadership and in reducing the spread of the disease in a number of countries including Brazil, India and South Africa. The report ends with a more optimistic statement, coming after barely 3 years of work. This second report is very much more didactic in its presentation compared to 1998, and appears to be targeting a more general audience. Piot's approach provides a collective analysis of the disease implying the importance of collective responsibility.

The report offers a clear definition of AIDS, discusses the response by the UN and then explains how UNAIDS works. It describes the many projects that UNAIDS has facilitated in various countries, on different issues ranging from leadership seminars to stigma-related activities through its work with the Global Business Council. It is an interesting document because it highlights how quickly and how broadly UNAIDS had become the face of the AIDS policy world in many contexts. The report also shows how a collective idea of AIDS came to established by the new programmes' perspective. While each of the projects mentioned in the report is located in its own socio-political context – ranging from Uganda to Argentina to Thailand, with many links to NGOs established – UNAIDS appears as the connection between the many different activities described. As a result, UNAIDS appears as the Global AIDS actor that gives coherence to the international response to AIDS. Gradually, the issue melds to offer an authoritative interpretation of the state of AIDS and the way in which this is made global through UNAIDS work.

This wide-ranging reach, which seems to link presidents of countries to local community workers and people living with HIV, builds the ground from which UNAIDS was able to speak with confidence in challenging the international system. In a joint report with the François-Xavier Bagnoud Center for Health and Human Rights at the Harvard School of Public Health, UNAIDS stated that

> Twenty years into the epidemic, AIDS is expanding three times faster than the funding to control it. In 1997, for example, donor nations plus the European Commission provided approximately US$ 150 million for HIV activities to African countries; at that time, there were some 21 million infected Africans and many more at risk. The report also indicates that after a quick influx of donor support, starting in 1990 the increase in annual AIDS funding began to slow (1999b: 30).

This report goes on to describe shortcomings in the funding regime and the weak allocation of resources in individual countries for AIDS. Again, it describes different kinds of HIV prevention and provides snapshot examples from different countries of what works and how. The report then describes how the objectives set out for UNAIDS have been operationalized. The reporting process thereby becomes a way of linking different countries, donors, people with HIV and a diverse set of interventions and interests into one global narrative. By publishing major reports such as these, UNAIDS not only fulfils its objectives and accounts for its work but also reasserts its position as the central actor in the global AIDS debate. There are also clear signs of the 'master discourse' within which AIDS is to be understood. Piot's first sentence in the 1999 report mentioned above establishes a moral challenge for the rest of the UN system. Later, under the heading *Why UNAIDS?* it is argued that,

> In 1986, the World Health Organization (WHO) had the lead responsibility on AIDS in the United Nations, helping countries to set up much-needed national AIDS programmes. But by the mid-1990s, it became clear that the relentless spread of HIV, and the epidemic's devastating impact on all aspects of human lives and on social and economic development, were creating an emergency that would require a greatly expanded United Nations effort (1999b: 11).

This not only frames the situation as an emergency but also positions UNAIDS as the key organization created to deal with it.[6] Here, the internal structure of UNAIDS as not only an international organization but also an organization that works with civil societies and people, becomes central to the way it justifies its position. Presenting the global state of AIDS as an emergency to which UNAIDS is leading the response, makes UNAIDS the custodian of AIDS consciousness in the international realm. And while the organization relies on funds from donors and co-sponsors and is not a funding organization, it has become the centre of attention by guiding how the epidemic should be tackled. Piot's words in the 1999 report and in subsequent reports are intentional guiding practices. They create the meaning of Global AIDS by framing how many people across the world face the disease and the challenges it presents in many different contexts.

This positioning also establishes a symbiotic relationship within the global AIDS community. The narrative of global AIDS as an emergency threat to all is built up around three central premises: first, the claims to medical authority that underpin UNAIDS guidelines, policy recommendations and more importantly, its monitoring role; second, the evaluation and reporting functions at country-level which provide an aggregate view of the state of Global AIDS; and third, on the basis of internal mechanisms that have enabled UNAIDS to develop a working relationship with civil society groups and organizations. In turn, these latter relationships have also enabled civil society groups to gain access to the international system which also brings funding possibilities to them. So supporting UNAIDS, becomes agreeing, at least publically, with its representation of AIDS as a global disease. These relationships are of material importance to UNAIDS, as they are central to its policy claims and legitimacy within the international organizational context. Here, we see the global community on AIDS projecting a unity towards outside publics via the agency of the UNAIDS, while internally relations are maintained through various

[6] Here, Piot appears to be 'speaking truth to power' (Hoppe 2011: 123). In this way, he locates UNAIDS both as an organization but also as the moral champion of the international AIDS community in relation to outside publics. This position becomes an ongoing feature of the organization's self-presentation during this early period of its work.

resource- and access-based considerations. In the meantime, global understanding of AIDS including how best to tackle the epidemic, is diffused through these relationships, including to the community level, in multiple socio-political settings through the policy practices of the different actors involved.

So in this sense the politics of global AIDS becomes a reflection of negotiations between actors differentially located within a community that presents itself as a particular relationship of actors relative both to one another and to the existing international system (Descombes 2014: 146). Gradually, and through these processes, UNAIDS came to present itself as the glue that holds this community together and, also, as the glue that maintains AIDS as a global problem within the international agenda. While indeed UNAIDS maintains the idea of the community with its leadership role, the actual relations that create the community are much more than just the sum total of the different actors included in UNAIDS' idea of the community.[7] The idea of the 'global problem' here in particular, allows UNAIDS in its self presentation to further underline the idea of there being a global community[8] comprising numerous actors' contribution to AIDS-related work becoming meaningful within this projected idea of Global AIDS.[9] Ultimately, the politics of Global AIDS is the outcome of these relationships and the way in which different actors utilize and facilitate the diffusion of idea concerning the global epidemic and its global community, within their work.

3.6 The Limits of UNAIDS and Change

When I talk about UNAIDS and its policies as a 'political' creation, I do so as an entry point to looking more closely at the system within which it functions. Once UNAIDS had been created, it expanded the political space within which HIV could be considered and the policies for intervention that could be developed. Both as an actor and as a space, it played a key role in communicating and creating guidelines for policy-making as well as implementation. One interesting example of this role lay in the preparation of guidelines on how one should use terminology such as 'HIV', 'AIDS' and compound phrases in relation to these terms, when writing (UNAIDS 2015c). UNAIDS terminological guidelines are now widely used by scholars and policy makers in the field. In a more directly policy-related area, its *Three Ones* policy framework aimed to provide a uniform structure through which

[7] This guiding towards mutual action or mutually comprehensible action is related to reframing the problem. In doing this, '[they] translate the new contextualised meanings into rules, norms and beliefs that infuse and unite a wider field of action' (Hoppe 2011: 165).

[8] The issue is not only conceptual but also guides shared action by all of those who become part of this community (Taylor 1971: 36).

[9] From the position of policy studies, the AIDS community can be seen comprising of actors 'institutionalized as oligopolistic policy subsystems' that are 'characterized by advocacy coalition politics, incremental analysis, problem-driven search and instrumental learning' (Hoppe 2011: 139).

global and local actors might coordinate their work in respect of HIV programme development and evaluation (UNAIDS 2004).

In most of UNAIDS activities the central concern was to keep AIDS on the international agenda and to disseminate particular knowledge and policies to develop a global framework. The latter also works as a support mechanism to achieve the former. Through its relations with a diversity of civil society actors and activists, including those who moved from different countries to work for the programme, UNAIDS succeeded in establishing itself as an international 'T-shirts and sandals' organization.[10] However, its image of being a civil society organization, or the AIDS community, was very much constrained by UNAIDS positioning within the international system.

This tension between organizational coordination and activism was an ongoing problem for a body which mirrored the politics of Global AIDS as it emerged at this juncture. While the programme used activist language to keep a global community on HIV together, what it could do in the field was limited by its policy and funding links with cosponsors, as well as by the international development aid modalities available. Inevitably over time UNAIDS has become too slow to engage for many civil society actors. However, it still provides an important space for civil society experts to gain access to the international system. Before discussing this further, it is important to look at one situation where this tension became very visible.

As I discussed above, even as late as the 1999 Annual report, UNAIDS seemed to argue that the treatment provision in developing countries was not a feasible option. In a rather non-committal manner that year's report stated that:

> In the industrialized world, where AIDS was identified almost two decades ago, treatment advances have led many people to assume that the epidemic is over. The facts tell us otherwise. New combination therapies have improved the quality of life and extended the survival of people with HIV, but they are far from a cure. The new antiretrovirals are expensive and often produce serious side effects. No one can predict how long their beneficial effects will last in a given patient, or how quickly the virus may mutate, becoming resistant to the drugs (1999b: 16).

The same document goes on to describe prevention success from various countries and broadly endorses behaviour change and prevention strategies for groups considered to be at risk. It is only in relation to discussion of mother-to-child transmission that treatment drugs are mentioned again

> … the UNAIDS Secretariat, UNICEF and WHO started planning concrete action to help countries translate the research into preventive action. Following negotiations with Glaxo Wellcome, the company made a donation of AZT and announced a substantial reduction in the price of the drug for the public sector of developing countries. This enabled planning to start on a major initiative for the reduction of mother-to-child transmission in 11 pilot countries (1999a, b, c: 38).

The report concludes with the argument that

[10] This image still pertains at many levels of UNAIDS. Staff moving from AIDS-related NGOs to UNAIDS and *vice versa* help maintain this appearance.

> As this report shows, the spread of HIV can be curtailed and the impact of AIDS alleviated. Countries everywhere need to base their response on policies known to be effective against AIDS – and setting these policies can take political courage. Countries also need financial resources to confront AIDS. It is now clear that the funding available comes nowhere near the real funding needs of the developing countries, which bear the brunt of over 90 % of the epidemic. For this global epidemic, solidarity is vital. Working together, it is possible to meet the challenges of AIDS (1999a, b, c: 51).

These 1999 discussions are important given that by this time the availability and efficacy of antiretroviral drugs in resource rich settings were well established. Also activism in these contexts made it clear that treatment needed to be placed centre-stage in policy interventions in the field. UNAIDS and its medical gaze might normally have agreed on this, but lack of resources and the inability to create resources independent of other international actors seems to have led to the situation outlined above. The official position promoted acknowledges the importance and relevance of treatment particularly in the case of mother-to-child transmission. However, it falls short of establishing treatment targets in resource poor settings. Some of the reasons given include the high cost of treatment and the non-availability of adequate medical infrastructure in resource-poor settings, particularly in Africa. Thus, arguably while UNAIDS became a global policy maker by establishing a global understanding of AIDS and by setting laying out key global policy frameworks, most of these were a function of what could have been done within existing resource allocations and power dynamics. A balancing act had been struck between being the leader of an international coalition constrained by existing resources, and a leading policy entrepreneur. More often it was the former that guided UNAIDS approach.[11]

One of the major challenges to this position emerged in the *Harvard Consensus Statement* published in 2001. Signed by many doctors, the document demonstrated step-by-step the importance of providing treatment in resource-poor settings and in Africa, particularly given the millions of people living with the HIV there. It argued

> Over the past two decades, the international response to HIV/AIDS in poor countries has emphasized HIV prevention, primarily due to the high cost of treatment and the limited resources available to developing countries. Despite this emphasis, the available scientific tools for prevention, in the absence of effective vaccines, remain inadequate to stop the spread of the disease. The very mention of AIDS treatment has often been avoided by donor agencies in wealthy countries, for fear that raised expectations would increase the financial and operational demands upon them, and detract from prevention efforts. The disparity in access to effective treatment between wealthy countries and developing countries is neither scientifically nor ethically justified at this time (2001: 4).

Four central reasons were provided as to why HIV prevention and treatment need to be considered together.

1. Treatment is essential to the 36 million people already infected with HIV, the vast majority of whom will die of AIDS without it;

[11] I qualify this statement by recognising that individuals working within the organization had their own personal links with civil society groups as well as policy advocacy networks. They were often engaged in informal discussion to generate reactions from these quarters to challenge the formal positions presented.

2. Treatment is necessary to optimize prevention efforts;
3. Treatment is necessary to save the children – and fabric – of societies;
4. Treatment is necessary for continuing economic development' (2001: 5).

This intervention in ongoing international policy discussion was important because it highlighted the limited way in which the international system was then thinking in global terms, worrying more about resources and distribution than the needs of people living (and dying) with HIV. This consensus statement was but one of a number of statements that not only established the feasibility of provision of HIV treatment globally, but also discussed possible targets for treatment roll-out.

While the medical community was establishing both technical and ethical justifications as to why it was imperative for the international community to provide treatment in Africa, in June 2001 the then Chief of United States Agency for Development, Andrew Natsios, provided the following justification as to why USAID was against such treatment.

> If we had [HIV medicines for Africa] today, we could not distribute them. We could not administer the program because we do not have the doctors, we do not have the roads, we do not have the cold chain… [Africans] do not know what watches and clocks are. They do not use western means for telling time. They use the sun. These drugs have to be administered during a certain sequence of time during the day and when you say take it at 10:00, people will say what do you mean by 10:00? (In America refusing to Save Africans: June 11, 2011 *New York Times*)

This statement in its sheer crassness generated a series of rebuttals. However, it also highlighted a major problem. USAID with all its resources was not interested in engaging with the HIV treatment debate and it was not the only international funding body that had concerns of this kind. For those of us doing research in Africa at that time, it was evident that the provision of treatment was a major concern. Working in Uganda and in Zambia, my personal recollection was of a policy of 'drugs for us and condoms for you'. Numerous civil society groups were frustrated by this, as were many people living with HIV. Voices raised in opposition showed clearly how local HIV community groups were gradually becoming part of a larger global network as they sought to influence the policy directions of international agencies such as USAID and UNAIDS.

Looking at the year 2010 UNAIDS report a decade later, the storyline one observes has dramatically changed. Not only does the report showcase a more confident organization but also it presents a different attitude towards the disease.[12]

[12]This change in directorship has represented for some a change in the way the organization engaged with itself and with HIV. Robin Gorna provides and important analysis of this change by reflecting on the new UNAIDS building in Geneva. She says 'it sent a strong message: the AIDS movement was here to stay… Strikingly at the start of 2009, a year after Michel Sidibé took over from Peter Piot as the new executive director…actual cracks started to appear in the new building. Much of the beautiful art was taken down…' (Gorna 2014: 107–08). Another view of this is offered in a discussion with a former staff member of UNAIDS, who said that UNAIDS was a knowledge organization and strong in research, now it is public relations focused, most of its work is on advocacy and not much on research.

Now under its second Executive Director Michele Sidibé, the 2010 UNAIDS report argues that

> Since 1999, the year in which it is thought that the epidemic peaked, globally, the number of new infections has fallen by 19 %. Of the estimated 15 million people living with HIV in low- and middle-income countries who need treatment today, 5.2 million have access—translating into fewer AIDS-related deaths. For the estimated 33.3 million people living with HIV after nearly 30 years into a very complex epidemic, the gains are real but still fragile. Future progress will depend heavily on the joint efforts of everyone involved in the HIV response (2010: 7).

1999–2000 proved to be a critical period in the way AIDS came to be established as a global problem. The early work of UNAIDS was vitally important in creating a broad-based community. The decision to include AIDS on the agenda of the UN Security Council of 10 January 2000 and the subsequent Security Council Resolution on the issue, brought home the importance of AIDS as a global problem. A parallel step was the inclusion of HIV-related targets to the Millennium Development goals in 2000, which placed the disease centre-stage in the international development agenda.

The AIDS community was further affirmed in its conviction of the importance of AIDS as a global concern by the special session of the UN General Assembly on HIV/AIDS held in New York in June 2001. This was an exceptional event as it brought many activists, people living with HIV and policy makers to New York to meet the world, as it were, at the UN headquarters. At the close of the event, the UN adopted a Declaration of Commitment, which listed challenges and achievements and set out timelines for achieving a step change in the global response, including in its Paragraph 55 a timeline for countries to develop strategies for HIV/AIDS treatment including the provision of anti-retroviral treatment (UN 2001 p.8). The declaration reinforced understanding of AIDS as a global problem that needed a global response and endorsed the leadership role of UNAIDS. It also affirmed the view of the disease and its global nature as developed by UNAIDS. The tone of declaration is similar in to that taken by Peter Piot in talking publicly about the disease as a global emergency where we know what to do, but we need global support (Piot 2001).

As emergencies require urgent action, the Declaration in paragraph 90 calls for the establishment of a global HIV/AIDS health fund. This is interesting as the same paragraph goes on to set as one of its objectives as to 'mobilize contributions to the fund from public and private sources with a special appeal to donor countries, foundations, the business community, including pharmaceutical (UN 2001: 14). The subsequent creation of the Global Fund to Fight AIDS, Tuberculosis and Malaria in 2002 reflects these concerns. It was established as a private foundation to receive funds from different donors that included governments, private sector and private foundations, and had the ability to distribute of these funds to countries in need in a more timely manner. The structure of the Global Fund was intended to be fast and flexible compared to international organizations, although it is important to note that many of the initial programmes developed and supported were created on the basis of the Global AIDS policy priorities and model interventions developed and disseminated through UNAIDS'.[13]

In the decade following 1999, treatment access became a global policy imperative. This was due to changes in the funding structures, including the emergence of the US President's Emergency Plan For AIDS Relief (PEPFAR),[14] in response to changing attitudes towards funding treatment, particularly in Africa. By 2003, UNAIDS was not only supporting and talking about treatment but had also launched a campaign, with its cosponsor WHO, entitled '3 by 5', which aimed to bring 3 million people into treatment by 2005.[15] According to Piot, speaking at the launch of the campaign, '[w]e must meet the challenge of expanding access to HIV treatment. This requires overcoming the formidable barrier of creating sufficient operational capacity – a key area where UNAIDS' Cosponsor, WHO, must play a critical role' (2003: 1). On the website outlining the campaign, it is stated that 'the problem is urgent as in poor countries 6 million people with HIV/AIDS need immediate ART' (WHO 2003: 1). This may be factually correct but the urgency had been there for some time, particularly after the effectiveness of ART had been established. Why was it that it was not until in 2003 that this urgency was recognised by the key global actors? This question is rhetorical, as the answer is obvious since UNAIDS was limited within its international position and while able to create a global community and play a leading role to keep the AIDS on the international agenda, it did not have the power to radically shift this agenda without the support of others. In this same period, when treatment became a central concern, prevention was decentred with funding shifting from it towards treatment-related activities. This change was evident for the many researchers who were in the field during this decade. Numerous interventions looking at prevention and behaviour change became unsustainable as a result of the way in which available resources were newly channelled into treatment-based interventions. While the 3 by 5 target was not realistic and was not met, treatment coverage did increase dramatically. However, there was yet another twist in the story.

The year 2010 UNAIDS report points to another important change that was gradually happening in this field. International financial support for global AIDS policies was levelling off. This was confirmed in following years when the need for treatment increased while funding remained at the same level. In a section of the 2010 report entitled *A New Vision*, it is argued that

> Fulfilling the UNAIDS vision of zero new infections will require a hard look at the societal structures, beliefs and value systems that present obstacles to effective HIV prevention efforts. Poverty, gender inequity, inequity in health and the education system, discrimination

[13] Here, I am observing the close relationship between UNAIDS and the Global Fund that reinforced the diffusion of a global vision on AIDS through projects and programmes development by national policy makers and civil society groups.

[14] PEPFAR was initially launched by G. W. Bush at his State of the Union address in 2003.

[15] There were other campaigns aimed to focus attention on AIDS designed by UNAIDS and its partners. These became mechanisms through which the AIDS community was brought together and reproduced itself as a global collective.

> against marginalized people, and unequal resource pathways all affect—and often slow—the HIV response. In a world that has had to learn to live with an evolving and seemingly unstoppable epidemic over the course of three decades, UNAIDS' vision of zero discrimination, zero new infections and zero AIDS-related deaths poses a challenge. But it is not a hopeless challenge. The vision of eliminating the toll that HIV imposes on human life can be made real using the knowledge and resources available today (2010: p.12).

This vision effectively makes UNAIDS a central organization to eradicate the disease. This position to a degree also extends the objectives and life of the organization until such a time as the disease is eradicated. Without doubt, throughout the 1990s and into the 2000s, UNAIDS has played an important role in developing and coordinating the global response, but it also became a very large organization in which many people are working.

3.7 Conclusion

These challenges and the impending end of the period marked by the Millennium Development goals were reflected on in a *Lancet* article in 2013 written by Sidibé and Kent Buse, who discuss the implications of these circumstances for the wider AIDS community. By way of concluding this chapter, I want to look briefly at their argument and its implications. After first pointing out that the AIDS response has been one of the most successful UN responses in the last 50 years, Sidibé and Buse argue that

> But we must recognise that the old ways of doing business are obsolete. The financial crisis has created funding constraints. Multilateralism is under pressure. Critical development issues contend for attention. A more ambitious global health agenda is increasingly focused on health rather than disease (2013a: 2148)

They then add that 'in forging a transformative governance architecture that will serve people best in 2020 and 2030 the principles that are fundamental to the success of the AIDS response must remain at the heart of the new agenda (2013a, b: 2148). Furthermore, they argue that 'whilst the AIDS community has a crucial role to play in forging the post-2015 we also need to listen, learn and identify areas for improvement (2013a: 2148).

This article is an important document because it appears to be written for the international development policy makers and donors on behalf of the AIDS community. At first sight, it appears reflexive and self-critical. It may even be seen as humble. It, nonetheless, proposes a particular way of thinking about the post-2015 governance of global health, arguing that

> the global health architecture needs no more than three agencies: one to handle financing; one to set norms and standards; and one for advocacy and accountability. An effective apex mechanism could bring different actors together, including the private sector (2013a: 2149).

The proposed framework is suspiciously similar to the global architecture and politics that developed around UNAIDS. In effect, in this article it seems UNAIDS is sending in its CV for the new job. This is perhaps not surprising given that the piece was written by the Executive Director of the UNAIDS and his then chief of Political Affairs and Strategy. They list a number of successes that might inform the future of global health, including the innovative organizational structure of UNAIDS and its various governance practices, involving civil society participation. The argument advanced is probably one of the clearest statements by the organization supporting my argument throughout this chapter that UNAIDS has created a community since 1996, and now stands ready to defend its position within the international system. By using the general language of AIDS and the AIDS community, the interest of the organization is to a degree refracted by this paper. The overall tone of the writing differs from that characteristic of UNAIDS' earlier framing of AIDS as an emergency requiring a health focus. However, towards the end of the article one of the last statements returns to the earlier prophetic voice, by pointing out that 'The AIDS movement is at a risky juncture. Any disinvestment in the response endangers the health MDGs and jeopardise returns on past investment' (2013a: 2149).

Another interesting aspect of this narrative is that the list of successes ascribed to the AIDS community is populated mostly by the activities of UNAIDS itself. The article provides evidence for the suggestion that there exists a question about the sustainability of AIDS interventions from within an emergency framework. The issue here is not whether this is about the survival of UNAIDS or not, the sustainability question is about the outcomes of polices that are seen as 'success' within the AIDS community on whose behalf the authors appear to speak. It is also curious that it is only at this late stage that UNAIDS appears willing to move beyond the emergency framing that had hitherto been deployed to great effect and which had produced the successes that are mentioned in the text. However, this frame has also created the circumstances within which a single disease focus dominated the policies and the implementation fields across the resource-poor settings: the prevalence of vertical interventions that have been created parallel to the exiting and mostly poor health systems in many countries have been the model of thinking. This discussion of an AIDS-centred global health model is an interesting idea, but UNAIDS will also have to engage with the question as to why such a logic has been so absent from the practices of the AIDS community to date. I will come back to this issue later in the book.

The evident reference to the collective as the AIDS 'community' in the article underwrites the existence of a global community. However, in this term it is not clear who exactly is part of this collective? Who speaks for them? The undifferentiated use of the idea of the AIDS community seems to include at the very least everyone living with HIV, all the others who are living with them, and the others who are trying to deal with their problems. The way in which the authors present their argument in terms of the achievements of this 'community', and by strong implication UNAIDS, suggests that the survival of the community is related to ongoing international support. This analysis lies at the centre of their AIDS-centric proposal. Their discussion also appears to suggest that the politics of Global AIDS is a function of the way in which the broader community participates within the international realm created through these organizational discussions. Their structural analysis suggests that the politics of Global AIDS has led to an upwards integration from the local to the international system. This kind of politics is of course somewhat distanced from the people living with HIV in diverse contexts. Peoples' experiences and understandings of AIDS become part of this considerations only after they have first been translated at the international level by UNAIDS using a Global AIDS lens.

So, in a paternalistic turn, the survival of UNAIDS and its network of relations is linked to the survival of the interventions that have been developed, and by extension to the survival of those who benefit from these interventions. In a sense, this is probably true given the vertical nature of many interventions that made them entirely reliant on external resources in many resource-poor settings. This view however is also about the dependence created in a system where political interests at the global level have only marginally diffused to the local political level, where support must be provided if interventions are to continue in the absence of international resources. In other words, the AIDS community itself is a manifestation of an order that was intended to function within the constraints of the international system. Thus, the meaning of the AIDS community here is not about UNAIDS *only* but it is also about the conceptual system UNAIDS facilitates through its engagement in public.

Chapter 4
Civil Society and Solidarity in the Politics of Global AIDS

The role played by civil society[1] activists and the space created by their activities in the emergence of the politics of AIDS is well established. Numerous activists, activist groups, community self-help groups and non-governmental organizations (NGOs) influenced debate and policy addressing AIDS as it emerged in early the 1980s. Civil society organisations have also had an important impact on the way in which the international system set about developing its response to AIDS. The specific governance structure created for UNAIDS, the policy modalities within which UNAIDS operates, and subsequently those of the Global Fund to Fight AIDS, Tuberculosis and Malaria, recognise the important role civil society actors play in this area. Today, the people-orientated language that informs the politics of Global AIDS reflects the continued significance and relevance of civil society organisations and solidarity for the future of Global AIDS debate (Smith et al. 2013).[2]

Given that much of this input derives from the activities of NGOs working with and serving people infected and affected by HIV in developing countries, it is essential to understand the kind of solidarity it currently represents. Sisonke Msimang in her introduction to a recent edited publication for the International HIV/AIDS Alliance provides a sobering account of the state of affairs when she identifies the gap between the *unfinished business* of AIDS in contrast to the publicly hopeful messages about the end of the disease one often reads. She argues that 'activists

[1] I broadly understand civil society as an arena of collective action organised around shared interests, purposes and values. Collective action can manifest itself in different spaces and in different associational and organizational forms. Although conventional theories often place civil society in opposition to the state (as the term 'non-governmental' suggests) as the central political domain, I think the notion of civil society should be widened to include the relationship to any political domain that is located superior to it in hierarchical socio-political relations (see de Tocqueville 2002; Edwards 2009; Gellner 1994).

[2] It is important to point out that while many speak about the international AIDS movement, the movement is heterogeneous and there are competing power dynamics within it. This heterogeneity is not only about different forms of activism but also about the nature of the issues engaged with by civil society.

H. Seckinelgin, *The Politics of Global AIDS*, Social Aspects of HIV 3,
DOI 10.1007/978-3-319-46013-0_4

who have forgotten how to fight are part of the problem. They are part of why there has not been sufficient strategic pushback against narrow, science-driven programmes and diminished funding in recent years' (2014: 6). Her evaluation and those of other contributors to the same volume link the decline in AIDS funding due to the 2008 economic crisis to a major change in the capacity of the AIDS organisations to have an impact. While I agree that this decline in funding has been important, I also think that the disempowerment of civil society has been gradually created by the way in which the contribution of civil society actors has been institutionalized in the politics of Global AIDS. Mark Heywood, in reflecting on AIDS activism in resource-poor settings, states that 'we [have] became enamoured with our own success, leading us to believe we had a power and ability to lift the response to HIV to ever greater heights – a power that, in fact we lacked' (2014: 17). As Msimang argues,

> ….. activists may have won important battles, but they often lost sight of the big picture. This meant that they retreated when they should have continued keeping up the pressure. Many activists incorrectly thought that the new fight would need to be taken to the boardrooms. While the ability to do this is crucial, sipping lattes and sharing PowerPoints will take us only so far. Activists who only speak the language of donors and international institutions are no longer activists: they become something else (2014: 5).

Both of these observations identify a critical issue within the Global AIDS framework, which has gradually institutionalized civil society action by setting limits on its horizons. It is this relationship between Global AIDS and its ability to incorporate and create uniformity for 'all' that has created the problem.

In this chapter, I will explore the implications of this transformation of civil society activity from an initial community activism which aimed to help each other, to a much more professionalized organizational activity that lobbies for political authority and desires to become an alternative policy implementer. The aim of looking at these transitions is to consider how they underwrote a major change in the way civil society was understood in relation to HIV, and then how this understanding came to influence the way in which civil society is framed in developing countries by international actors including international NGOs. These steps allow me to consider how far the ethos of solidarity, often discussed in the literature as being broadly based on the AIDS activism of the 1980s, relates to the circumstances in which many groups currently work in resource-poor settings.

4.1 Emergence of AIDS Activism and Civil Society Organizations

It was in countries such as the USA that civil society confrontation with the political system first marked the beginnings of the politics of AIDS. With time, this civil society experience, with its tools of public activism, has become an implicit model for others to use within the global AIDS system. The early demands of many activists in the USA were about health systems including medical research, drug development and care systems to address their health needs. While these demands clearly politicized medicine, they also medicalized the nature of AIDS debate in the long run. Given that people living with HIV did not have access to the health and other resources to deal with AIDS, they turned debate on its head to claim their health rights as citizens. The critical point here is that their actions were underpinned by an already existing system of rights, including freedom of speech and association, which regulated the nature of these confrontations. Even if there was a confrontation with political authority and a major challenge took place, people still had the political and legal rights to have that debate. In James Holston's view, this situation already indicates an underlying 'citizen's sense of [an] objective source of right in citizenship entails a corresponding sense of subjective power- power to change existing arrangements' (2009:252). The activist process shows that this confrontation was about redefining the belonging of people in a system that was obliged to respond to their needs, as opposed to allowing such people to be framed as outside its socio-political interests. So, here we can observe two interlocking moves. On the one hand there was a real resource issue in the face of the epidemic that needed to be addressed, while on the other hand addressing it also meant that the state had to change its approach to engaging with particular categories of people (those living with and affected by HIV) over time.

One way of looking at this is to use Sarah Schulman's (2013) framing. Reflecting on her experience as a long time AIDS activist, she considers where activism in the USA is today. She argues that for analytical clarity one needs to distinguish between 'the AIDS of the past and ongoing AIDS' (2013:42). She maintains that 'neither is over, although they are treated quite differently in the present moment' (2013: 42). The distinction here is about the way in which AIDS came to be tackled in the 1980s and the way it is framed today. She argues that the impact of the former has been very important on the present, but that *ongoing AIDS* has produced a different kind of engagement. She identifies ongoing AIDS as being 'both maintained and addressed by globalization – a sort of worldwide gentrification in which specificity of experience, understanding, and need are glossed over by a homogenized corporate net…' (2013:42). She then adds that '[m]arketed as "AIDS in Africa" ongoing international AIDS has inspired a kind of insipid charity mentality in the citizen who expresses her opinions through the products she consumes' (2013:43). In the USA, up until the present, she argues that

> [w]hile death rates have declined domestically, infection rates are increasing. The failure of US prevention programs to raise percentage of effectiveness gets addressed with the gentrified cure-all: marketing…Offering young men of colour free Metro cards to come to "prevention counselling" does not change the fact that they are economically, politically and representationally pushed aside. But the larger problems – the United States' refusal to destigmatize and integrate gay people on our own terms, treat drug users effectively, support reasonable public education, provide health care, and stop incarcerating Black males-these policies are what keep infection rates high (2013:43–44).

This perspective provides important insight into the way in which the civil society debate has changed over time. It broadly traces a move from community activism based on people themselves and their work within their own communities, towards a more generalized framing organised around professionalism and charity.[3] There has been a parallel shift from hyper-political and confrontational activist engagement to a much more technical and professionalized encounter within the organizational context of the policy process. Accompanying this there has been a move from demanding recognition and rights to thinking about how best to deliver health and social services. While there can be little doubt that by participating in the policy process many activists have confronted the political conservatism inherent within the policy making in general, their participation has given rise to a gradual professionalization around the particular technical questions relevant to different HIV-related civil society groups. Schulmann describes this situation as on in which 'activists win policy changes and bureaucracies implement them' (2013:12).

The extract above is also revealing because it points out that while AIDS activism in the USA managed to become a formal part of policy discussions and processes, this has had a limited impact, for instance, on the life circumstances of Hispanic and African Americans, compared to other groups.[4] The relationship between this outcome and the move from activism towards professionalization as a system of engagement for civil society bears critical examination. While success made it possible for civil society actors to participate in the HIV policy process, the activist outlook was transformed into technical expertise and service delivery within an existing system of class and race based prejudices and exclusions.

Considered from Rancière's perspective on politics, there can be no doubt that AIDS activism throughout 1980s reflected a 'dissensual subjectification that reveals the difference of a society itself' (2010: 42). Activism pointed to the need to acknowledge difference and through this to address rights claims. However, by doing this particular racial and class based distinctions within the broader social order were replicated. Raymond A. Smith, Richard G. Parker, Jonathan Garcia and Robert H Remien argue that

> ..... [the] middle class, white, and often well-educated gay men who have been the "ground zero" of HIV/AIDS in the developed world were able to bring resources to bear that other marginalized groups might not be able to, including financial contributions, professional

[3] The initial civil society response to AIDS in the USA was based on a strong solidarity among infected and affected communities to support each other as reflected in 'the creation of Gay Men's Health Crisis (GMHC) and the People with AIDS Coalition (PWAC) and in early 1990s through the pioneering work of the AIDS Coalition to Unleash Power (ACT UP)' (Smith 2013:13). Here Cohen's observation of the initial emergence of activism in the USA among urban middle-class white gay men provides important insight into the ways in which solidarity for political action replicated class distinctions via a paternalistic solidarity for gay men from different backgrounds (1998).

[4] The 2012 International AIDS Conference in Washington DC revealed the gap between differences in HIV-related experience in this regard within the USA. A rally on the mall before the opening of the conference, which aimed to show civil society solidarity, was a significant event. It was dominated by African-American participants and their needs while also many street signs in the city centre were targeting condom use among African-American men. The gravity of the situation for members of this particular population can be seen in the special issue of *The Lancet* (July 2012) launched at the conference.

> skills, "cultural capital" in the creative professions and, to some extent, influential social network (2013:29).

This observation is important because while it reveals the nature of the solidarity that first motivated activism, it also points to the seeds of differentiation within the initial solidarity movement. With time, this differentiation has become more important as solidarity has become more professionalized and has transformed itself into a charity-based, more paternalistic, civil society activity. This transformation is about a bifurcation between those who can participate in policy networks as the professional voices of community representing those who cannot, and those who gradually become the patients or clients of the policies developed and implemented by AIDS NGOs. The above statement identifies the critical characteristics of the activists who were able to assume the role of speaking for themselves and on behalf of others. Although the solidarity movement and its impact are often presented through the ability of the activist to turn their personal experience of HIV into policy-relevant knowledge, this impact was also facilitated by the above-mentioned social characteristics. This nuanced relationship assumed a differentiated sense of 'belonging' within the broader society, and underlies why some can and some cannot participate in these discussions. Given these conditions, the success of the solidarity movement was about using a particular strategy to create a group identity organised around HIV independent of individual differences, to demand access to health resources and to target the disease independent of whoever got it.[5]

This solidarity-driven tactical representational politics created both a move towards the professionalization of civil society actors and a process within which internal differences were obscured for the benefit of having a stronger voice in access to policy processes (Halperin 2014). Without doubt, many who worked in these increasingly professionalized organizations were members of different communities infected and/or affected by HIV. These personal links enabled the presence of solidarity within the overall process. But this also changed over time. While the language of solidarity has remained, the nature of experience-based solidarity has gradually disappeared.

There have been several outcomes of this process. For instance, the success of this particular kind of civil society activity can be observed in the fact that some civil society actors, as brokers, participate in policy debate by making HIV central to policy discussions. The relationship between this professionalized civil society participation in HIV-related policy making and the outcomes of these policies for particular groups remains mostly unarticulated however. The relationship between local grass-roots activism and professional civil society organizations is recognized as central within the HIV sector and gives rise to inclusion through consultative processes. There are numerous workshops and conferences in which professional activists and activist-scientists meet communities. These are typically designed as two-way communication processes in which communities are informed about new

[5] This can also be read from Cohen's class-based analysis as an attempt to reproduce middle-class privilege that was challenged by association with a gay disease, thus reflecting a particular view both on the sexuality and the experience of the disease (1998).

policy changes or initiatives, while professionals 'listen' to community views. These events also create a stage on which to perform community solidarity – both for the benefit of people living with HIV and also for other policy actors. The overall point here is that the drive to maintain links with the grass-roots points to the survival of an abstract idea of solidarity. But, there is a growing gap between activists working at the grass-roots in particular communities and those civil society organizations and their networks that set the national agenda by participating in national and international policy making processes.

Furthermore, the fact that this relational-pattern is replicated, both at national and international levels, indicates the importance of the link between civil society groups and international policy makers for the public legitimacy of those AIDS organizations working within the Global AIDS context. It allows them to make claims to represent people's voices to partake in debates over scarce resource allocation.

4.2 Is It the Same Civil Society We Are Talking About in Resource-Poor Settings?

Gay and lesbian communities were central to community activism in both North America and Western Europe.[6] Gay community activism around AIDS created the political momentum to address the needs of people living with HIV. It gave rise to a form of social mobilization generated by particularly disadvantaged groups and their claim to resources on the basis of their citizenship rights. In this sense, the activism of this period fits well with the definition of contentious politics offered by Tilly and Tarrow (2006), laying the foundations for the civil society response later in the epidemic (Altman 1994; Epstein 1996; Treichler 1999). Numerous activist groups developed technologies of protest to engage with the public authorities through repertoires of protest that emerged across multiple locations (see Aggleton et al. 1997; Brown 1997; Gould 2009). Many of the strategies developed and first used within the USA later became globally implemented policy tools for entry into first national, and then international, policy debate. In this process, civil society over time both in the USA and in Western Europe transformed itself into a professional and political actor.[7] However, this transformation did not preclude the existence of different kinds of more direct activism surviving in different contexts.

---

[6] I focus on these areas in particular because their links with the institutionalization of activism in the emerging politics of Global AIDS through the formation of new AIDS organizations was important. I also recognize that there were dynamic and influential local civil society actors in a number of different countries including Australia, Brazil, Thailand and India (Biehl 2009; Parker 2009; de la Dehesa and Mukherjea 2012; Power 2015).

[7] This change can be also measured by considering the situation from a generic civil society perspective of looking at the volume of all non-governmental activity on AIDS in the US or internationally. This is not helpful. This approach does not say much about the nature or content of the activity or how it has changed over time.

Randy Shilts' observations of the 4th International AIDS conference in 12 June 1988 in Stockholm highlight the direction of change emerging as early as the late 1980s. He writes that,

> [T]he opening ceremony of the AIDS conference demonstrated the extent to which the epidemic had become not only respectable, but wholly institutionalized. Between elegant music and solemn first speeches, the evening was more like [PBS special] than a scientific conference. The senior statesmen of AIDS research Drs Robert Gallo and Luc Montagnier delivered the opening scientific addresses. Neither researcher had much new to offer, but their speeches were now part of AIDS conference ritual' (1988: 612page).

He goes on to argue that, '[w]ith the growing international AIDS network the catch-word of the 1988 conference became the 'institutionalization' of AIDS. Indeed, the Stockholm AIDS conference launched an International AIDS Society with Dr Paul Volberding as its president-elect' (1988: 612–613). Via this process, medical scientists as activists came to occupy centre stage, with the International AIDS Society (IAS) becoming 'the representative of the international scientific community and often the voice of reason in controversies that have plagued the response to the epidemic' (Kallings and McClure 2008: 6). While dynamic grassroots civil society on AIDS still took place, particularly in resource-rich settings, the nature of civil society engagement with the epidemic changed dramatically in some of the poorer parts of the world. Gordenker et al., write

> ….. as consciousness of AIDS grew, new ASO [AIDS service organizations] and AIDS-related NGOs mushroomed in various parts of the Western world and to a much lesser extent and unevenly in developing regions…Public agencies usually were reluctant to channel funds to these newly formed organizations, largely because of uncertainty as to their capacity, not to speak of their approaches…For different reasons, nearly all AIDS-related NGOs were so poorly financed that their ability to provide care or to put pressure on public agencies were restricted. Moreover, a wide spectrum of NGOs feared that accepting government funding would jeopardize their credibility in the eyes of their clients (1995: 92).

As they worked to participate in policy debate, civil society groups needed to show both competence in the subject matter and legitimacy in relation to the groups they claimed to represent. They also needed funding to be able to participate in the policy making process. In order to move from activism and self-help to being heard by policy making actors, many organisations became NGOs. The number of NGOs working on AIDS in resource-poor settings mushroomed, creating an area that is now considered a sector itself: namely, the 'HIV/AIDS sector'. The international policy frameworks that developed in the late 1990s and in the early 2000s required NGOs and other civil society groups (including community groups and self-help organizations), to become part of the funding relationship between international funders and resource-poor countries.

The organizational intensity and the public visibility of HIV-related NGOs are now considered indicators of success. The presence of these organizations is seen as representing the claims and demands of people living with HIV within the formal policy processes. This indicates both a major shift in the attitudes of policy makers towards NGOs as actors of policy implementation, particularly in the resource poor settings, and in the attitudes of NGOs as civil society actors in these contexts towards international funders and the policy makers who broadly finance them. What can be observed here is a transformation in civil society activity from grassroots activism to professionalization and institutionalization via the route of *having a seat at the table*, receiving funding at the international level and, finally, by becoming models to inform civil society activity in resource-poor settings.

There is an intimate relationship between the emerging Global AIDS view on NGOs and the broadly neo-liberal international policy frameworks that have tended to view civil society or NGOs as 'partners' to whom to contract out social services that were traditionally delivered by the state (Brown 2015). There is also a relationship between the expansion of this position among major international development aid donors, particularly throughout the late 1980s and the 1990s, and the growth of HIV-related NGOs in this period (Seckinelgin 2002; Nair 2013). In addition to the role of international funders such as the World Bank, private foundations such as the Ford and MacArthur Foundations early on, and later the Gates Foundation, also helped in this process by funding the emergence of widespread civil society activity on AIDS based mostly on the work of NGOs across the world (Harman 2010; McGoey 2015).[8] The key analytic issue here is the relationship between the AIDS activism of the 1980s and its impact on policy thinking, and policy processes inherent in the emergent international politics of AIDS. A particular form of activism came to be institutionalized within international organizations further motivating the emergence of a professionalized civil society sphere in resource poor-settings. I argue that this process highlights the transformation of politics from activists partaking in politics of change to activists partaking in the Global AIDS sphere as organizational representatives to benefit from resource relations. Throughout this process, the politics of Global AIDS concerns the way in which international actors frame the understanding of the problem and reproduce this understanding by including other actors in the global process (through solidarity to deal with HIV as an emergency); set up the priorities for other participants to follow in the global AIDS sphere (coordination through policy priorities) and; and c) then develop the policy modalities to be used by all actors agreeing with these priorities (co-option through policy participation) (Seckinelgin 2009a).[9]

[8] Arguably these interventions shared a common set of assumptions about the role of civil society that is familiar within US political culture, where community self-help groups are considered to be the backbone of the social make up (Seckinelgin 2002).

[9] Overall, this suggests a 'process in which knowledge about policies, administrative arrangements, institutions in one time and/or place is used in the development of [these] in another time and/or place[s]'(Dolowitz and Marsh 1996): 344).

4.3 The Modality of Civil Society Professionalization and Its Transformation

The transformation of grass-roots activism into more professionalized forms has informed how AIDS-related civil society activism has been incorporated in international policy circles. The policy practices of both WHO's GPA and later UNAIDS facilitated the progressive inclusion of ever more professionalized civil society groups in international debate. As a result, civil society's role as a policy partner has become an established global policy modality. This approach was based on the experiences of both particular policy makers in the USA and Western Europe and the way in which some local AIDS activists moved to work within the international policy arena, bringing their own experiences to bear on activism for policy intervention in a different context.

One important illustration of this move from the local to the international can be observed in the Denver Principles of 1983. This was an early self-empowerment declaration by people with HIV seeking to claim their agency in the face of the epidemic. The Principles boldly announced that 'we condemn attempts to label us "victims", a term which implies defeat, and we are occasionally patients, a term which implies passivity, helplessness and dependence of the care of others. We are people with "AIDS"'(1983: 1). These demands framed later AIDS debate by establishing the centrality of the rights of HIV positive people to be part of the fight against AIDS. This rights-based position came to be internationalized at the Paris AIDS Summit in 1994 where 42 countries indicated agreement to the principle of the Greater Involvement of People Living with HIV (GIPA) in the policy process – from inception to implementation and monitoring – to improve the relevance, acceptability and effectiveness of HIV-related policies. UNAIDS later adopted this principle as part of its overall approach.

> Within organizations, the participation of people living with HIV can change perceptions, as well as provide valuable experiences and knowledge. At the community and social levels, public involvement of people living with HIV can break down fear and prejudice by showing the faces of people living with HIV and demonstrating that they are productive members of, and contributors to, society. (UNAIDS 1999c:1)

This action can be seen as part of a larger process of aligning rights-based claims within UNAIDS work, such as in 1998 when the Office of the United Nations High Commissioner on Human Rights and UNAIDS published the *International Guidelines on HIV and Human Rights*. However, in much of UNAIDS work a trade-off between human rights and technical intentions has remained.[10] In this context, civil society organisations may participate in AIDS related policy debates but access

[10] This trade-off can also be seen more generally in terms of how treatment access and rights-based health approaches remain unreconciled in a context where pharmaceutical interests still predominate. See recent work by Obijiofor Aginam and John Harrington (2013).

to resources based on rights, and the rights of the marginalized, remains more difficult to achieve.[11]

One interesting insight into the existence of this trade-off between the two positions is reflected in Mark Heywood's comment that

> ….. between 2006 and 2012 I was the chairperson of the UNAIDS Reference Group on HIV and Human Rights. Unfortunately, one thing that struck me throughout my tenure was how little the UNAIDS senior management understood of human rights and how poorly they paid attention to the recommendations of the reference group' (2014:18).

Significantly, the internationalization of a particular kind of advocacy work through capacity-building workshops and seminars motivated, for instance, the creation of groups of HIV positive people in many different locations across the world. This was done in the expectation that these groups would both support one other and take advocacy leadership within their societies to address HIV-related concerns. Through these processes, both Global AIDS priorities (for coordination) and shared tools of engagement (co-option) have been transferred – including *coming out* as an HIV positive person and talking about it publically to increase public visibility. According to Vinh-Kim Nguyen this kind of 'confessional politics' may be seen as an attempt to create alternative domain for citizenship rights: '[b]eing HIV positive, in this context, constituted a kind of parallel and derivative citizenship. Clinic ID cards provided access to treatment and health-life itself' (2010:112). Such an approach has gradually come to reference agency on the basis of an individual's HIV status to resource relations outside their own socio-political context.

In many resource-poor settings, civil society organisations hitherto lacked the political agency or knowledge to advance the kinds of interventions required to deal with AIDS. International actors recognized the need to encourage particular kinds of civil society practices to engage with AIDS. Thus, policy interventions such as the establishment of HIV positive people' groups have aimed to stimulate civil society activity. Such groups have also been used to build a broader solidarity that could then be used to coordinate what needs to be done at the grassroots level. The organizational modality of this kind of grassroots' activity reflects a particular US political experience, which seeks to establish a more general model of action framed by partnership between civil society and the political authority to deal with AIDS. Viewed another way, this represents an attempt to establish an 'agent of transfer' who can engage with Global AIDS and localize their policies (Evans and Davies 1999: 366). This approach eventually turned local civil society activity into 'project outputs' for international NGOs and experts to highlight NGOs' own impact on the world, and thus to register their participation in Global AIDS.

One significant example of this was the creation of the International HIV/AIDS Alliance in 1993 as a civil society umbrella organization funded by a number of international/national donors to stimulate and support community work across a

---

[11] This situation was of course noticed by international policy actors such as UNAIDS and IAS leading them to use the AIDS 2010 XVIII International AIDS Conference in Vienna to focus on the relationship between human rights and AIDS under the conference banner of *Rights Here, Right Now.*

number of countries. The original team included a number of first generation North American AIDS activists. At the time of writing, the Alliance works in 40 countries supporting many community-based interventions. Another example was the creation of the Multi-country HIV/AIDS Programme for Africa (MAP) by the World Bank in 1999, which expended over 2 billion USD in a decade. While this level of financing is significant in that it creates dependence at the local level, the organizational impact of this initiative in motivating the creation of National AIDS Councils (NACs) as a condition for funding was more important. NACs were to be multi-stakeholder structures to coordinate the national response and engage with donors and global policy actors, and by design had to include civil society groups. This modality later turned into the 2004 UNAIDS policy of the *Three Ones*, which further institutionalized the World Bank's modality of AIDS-related work in non-African contexts. The Global Fund to Fight AIDS, Tuberculosis and Malaria, through its the Country Coordinating Mechanism (CCM), which was designed to develop projects before their submission for financial support, also required country-wide consultation and civil society organizations were again included as part of these processes. Two other approaches in the 2000s further advanced the development of civil society based on the NGO sector. The US President's Emergency Plan For AIDS Relief from its inception in 2003 motivated the further inclusion and expansion of NGO sector because its funding targeted immediate needs such as treatment delivery (Coutinho et al. 2012; AIDS 2014a). In 2003, the Gates Foundation funded a number of large structural interventions such as AVAHAN project in India for service-delivery involving treatment, again heavily reliant upon civil society participation (Bonnel et al. 2013: 59).

Throughout these processes, particular activist experiences were transformed into generic relationships between activists and society through their institutionalization in projects as local NGO activities. In the transfer, civil society experiences were homogenised with observed success being associated with the quality of civil society action in general. Such an input orientation, which considers creating the right kind of organization as central to producing the expected results, civil society activism is reduced to its organizational aspects (Scharpf 1999; Rothstein 2009; Crozier 2010). This sets the successful creation of organizations as the outcome measure, rather than what is actually done to influence change. To be able to participate in Global AIDS, local organizations have to show their 'relationship capacity', that is their ability to work with global actors within the already established AIDS modalities (Castells 2009:34). Once this capacity is recognized or established by expert workshops on capacity building, local civil societies can become more integrated into the Global AIDS system.

Throughout this process, various issues are sidelined or ignored. These include how politics, as the partaking that underwrote the Denver Principles, has been reduced to a utilitarian modality to facilitate global actors' implementation strategies. Beyond this, the context within which initial success was observed is ignored and the temporality of this success is discounted, with the ability to deliver 'results' being assumed to be an inherent characteristic of all civil society organizations.[12] Additionally, class, race, cultural and professional biases in civil society, leading to the problems identified by Schulman in relation to the experiences of African-American people, are not taken into account. Finally, one of the central lessons of history is ignored: while civil society organisations may provide alternative thinking and action, they also carry with them their own interests and the biases and prejudices of the broader society within which they function.

4.3.1 The Implications of Becoming a Broker

Given the way in which Global AIDS has developed, civil society's role internationally turns political contestation based on the right to resources and recognition into a professional activity undertaken by NGOs with technical expertise in service delivery. Civil society participation thereby becomes a policy implementation modality.[13] This is not incidental given the reluctance of many governments to engage directly with AIDS and the lack of legal and political guarantees that make civil society activism possible. Related to this, there has been an explicitly political agenda in the development of Global AIDS. International policy actors have wanted gradually to create a domestic political dynamic to change the conditions that frame the experiences of people living with HIV. The aspiration was that the many technical interventions that required NGOs to be part of the policy process would in turn lead to the development of more dynamic civil society processes. International support attempted both to help communities that were struggling with AIDS but at the same time to engineer the emergence of a civil society response around HIV. However, rather than this being led by civil society activism itself, as had been the case in North America and Western Europe, the process was reversed by supporting the assumed conditions for activism in resource-poor settings through funding to 'grassroots' organizations. International policy interventions sidestepped the thorny politics of this stance by making their approach seem technical. By focusing on globally framed interventions that appeared technical, international agencies limited the horizons and agency of local groups to set their own agendas within particular socio-political settings. Beyond this, the imbalanced availability of expert knowledge and resources within Global AIDS created a critical dependence of civil society

[12] Similar claims to use the civil society response to HIV in Brazil as a model for other contexts have been challenged. Berkman et al. (2005) argue that success cannot be considered as a generic outcome beyond the particular socio-political context in which it emerges. In the case of Brazil, this implies particular ways of engaging with citizenship through social solidarity.

[13] The professionalization of activism has been well observed by Alicia Garza, a leader of *Black Lives Matter*, in an interview reflecting on her social justice work as a queer African-American activist. She states that 'San Francisco broke my heart over and over. White progressives would actually argue with us about their right to determine what was best for communities they never had live in' (Cobb 2016: 35). The implications of this are relevant for international 'solidarity' and civil society claims to implement rights-based policies.

groups on international experts and funding. So, while it was within the dissemination of knowledge and funding that generic policy targets and policy modalities were set, this process established an agency for civil society groups that was limited to the Global AIDS community.

For instance, the implementation of GIPA principles can be seen as somewhat tokenistic. The inclusion of people with HIV remains a representational tool by not providing the resources for them to have actual impact on these processes. This kind of partaking, or perhaps better 'co-option', allows public visibility but has limited impact on the general direction of Global AIDS thinking. In the late 2000s, recognition of this fact created debate about MIPA, or the *Meaningful* Involvement of People Living with HIV, as a way of getting global actors to think more carefully about their commitments (Safaids 2016).

It is also important to recognise how Global AIDS-related civil society processes came didactically to be constructed by international AIDS experts with activist backgrounds from elsewhere. The approach generated numerous guidelines and best practice documents propagating particular strategies and tools to be used to build community mobilization and solidarity, for example. These aimed to get different groups to replicate what needs to happen, as already articulated by the Global AIDS institutions. As result, management through Best Practice, such as by faithful adherence to UNAIDS guidelines, turned activism into a practice focusing on replicating ways of doing AIDS work so as to show results in line with the targets set by the Global AIDS agenda – implying a move from partaking in rights claims to partaking in order to comply with policy delivery mechanisms. Combined with the resource relations and the hierarchical claims on expertise to deal with AIDS, civil society groups have emerged in many resource-poor settings, particularly in Africa, not to lead any overtly 'political' challenge, but to apply international expertise and technical skills to advocacy and service delivery.

In time, many interventions motivated the creation of many local organizations. As global priorities changed, Global AIDS actors also responded to the demands from the AIDS-related NGOs they had created for further resources and funding. In this process, and through their work as 'brokers', NGOs have diffused global actors' AIDS-specific policy thinking detailing externally determined policy priorities for resource-poor settings. This has often been done paying lip service to issues such as human rights, gender and poverty-related concerns. In most cases, resources have been delivered as vertical interventions paralleling existing health and social policy frameworks in resource-poor settings. All too frequently, international NGOs from elsewhere in the world have been tasked to carry out the required implementation.

Today it might be possible to argue that circumstances have changed in many resource-poor settings and it is possible to talk about home-grown activism together with home-grown NGO sectors. However, it is important to consider what is meant by 'home grown' within this context. While it is undeniable that there are many places where we can see activist groups, AIDS service organizations and NGOs working in the field, I agree with Mark Heywood in his reflections on the pre-2008 successes of civil society activism, which placed AIDS in the international policy agenda and influenced the emergence of new funding architecture for establishing antiretroviral treatment as a global policy issue (2014:14–17). The key issue here is about how this form of activism and its agency to influence can be made sustainable and able to survive without international support.

A number of people have argued that this form of analysis may be too uniform in its treatment of resource-poor settings and that there are major differences among many countries and their civil society spheres (Lewis 2014; Knutsson 2016). I agree there are differences between nations. However, even when these differences taken into account, the funding generated and the space opened up by the politics of Global AIDS have been pre-eminent sources of support for activism in resource poor settings.[14] There are a number of issues here. First, many national governments have agreed to work with these structures and to recognize the role of their own AIDS-specific civil society groups in this field. Second, given that these organizations were bringing with them resources, local governments have been keen to collaborate.[15] Third, over time HIV-related civil society activity has become progressively fragmented between those who have a voice in these internationally-led processes and those who excluded from this. Finally, through the availability of resources facilitated by having access to civil society organizations, people have encountered the effects of Global AIDS policy for a long time in clinics, offices or simply the HIV-related projects run by NGOs in many contexts.

4.3.2 Rethinking an Advocacy Modality

One commonly used theoretical approach to justify the close relationship between local NGOs and international actors and networks is provided by Margaret E. Keck and Kathryn Sikkink's *boomerang effect* theory of international advocacy (1998). The argument here is that it is important for local groups to work with international organizations that can provide support to advocate domestically for socio-political change. One issue, that is particularly relevant for HIV-related work in developing countries, is missed here. It is one thing to provide justification for international policy makers' approach to civil society in general, but it is something else to consider the nature of sustainable civil society work within a given context. Keck and Sikkink's work is interesting but it focuses on advocacy outcomes as instances of

[14] Many would point to domestic activism on AIDS in Brazil, India, and South Africa and in Thailand. However, these countries do not present typical socio-political conditions for resource-poor settings in general. Furthermore, the changes witnessed in these contexts also bear witness to the relationship between these countries and the broader policy considerations within the global process. For instance, Joao Biehl's (2009) work traces reveals the impact of broader neo-liberal policies on HIV and on the experiences of people living with HIV in Brazil (2009). In a similar vein, it is hard to take domestic activism on HIV in South Africa as representative of possibilities in all southern African countries. South Africa presents us with a particular pattern politics of solidarity and awareness of rights due to its history.

[15] For instance, according to Tim Hildebrandt's (2011) work, even in China regional bureaucracies have considered international AIDS funding as a way of attracting resources into their region.

success, rather than thinking about change and sustainability in what is achieved over time. They focus on agenda setting and not on how a set agenda comes to be actively implemented for change. The sustainability of AIDS-related civil society work and its ability to initiate socio-political challenges to influence change beyond internationally developed policy programmes depends on the capacity of local actors to have agency within their own societies.[16] It is clear that local NGOs are very much at the centre of Global AIDS relief work and that this activity is possible due to international support. However, it is not as clear how NGOs, without the material resources being provided, can initiate socio-political debate in their local context beyond the priorities set by Global AIDS institutions. Will many of these NGOs survive in such a way that their work is sustainable? This is not simply a question of recognizing the resource dependency of civil society groups in delivering their work, it is also about considering the sustainability of what is being done in people's lives and the capacity and agency of local groups to decide their own agenda outside the policy directions provided by Global AIDS actors. The last point is central. Many local actors that are part of the Global AIDS picture have only a very limited role in deciding the best approach to deal with the HIV-related needs in their own contexts (see Qureshi 2015). Often, the community empowerment and capacity-building programmes supported by international actors to develop the capacity of local groups are in line not with local knowledge and experience, but with Best Practice guidelines emanating from global policy fora.

4.4 Civil Society Practices Within Global AIDS Spaces

There are different ways of thinking about how civil society practices are brought into alignment with Global AIDS processes. In the analysis above, I have talked of *creation* (to deal with the lack of local activism and the absence of organizational forms), *coordination* (dealing with the problems of expansion of groups, inefficiencies concerning the distribution of limited resources, and the implementation of particular ways of dealing with AIDS) and *co-option* (turning local groups into service delivery and implementation agencies) as dominant forms. In addition to these processes, which produce and reproduce particular civil society practices in line with the Global AIDS framework, another important issue is the solidarity that must be created. Through its performance, global solidarity legitimates Global AIDS policy intervention. Solidarity serves as an internal legitimacy mechanism in the global AIDS community in addition to being a representational communication strategy for the outside world to show the unity of the AIDS community and the existence of a global movement.[17] These are interlinked coordination and co-option

[16] An important analysis of this particular issue has been developed by Ulla Pape (2014) in her study of the way in which the NGO sector has developed in response to AIDS in Russia.

[17] This is also about a social movement strategy to show the worthiness of the cause to the general public along with the diversity and numbers of people supporting that cause (Tilly 2004).

processes that maintain the relations between key global actors and civil society groups at multiple levels. The volume and the style of these policy relations provide evidence of the solidarity and the existence of the global AIDS movement.

These coordination and co-option processes can be observed as new policy directions come to influence the practices of many NGOs across the world, through the implementation of what appears to be similar policies on prevention, care or treatment. These changes may sometimes be on substantive policy issues (such as the change from focusing on HIV prevention to treatment, or to the claimed importance of voluntary medical male circumcision) but sometimes they are about the diffusion of policy categories (targeting orphans, women and MSM) that are used for targeting. These changes also underlie the resource dependency of local organizations and the way this impacts on their own agency to decide what to do.

In the early 2000s, while conducting research in central East Africa, I encountered many international NGOs that were working with local groups. At the time, these were mostly interested in setting up Voluntary Counselling and Testing (VCT) clinics in rural communities. The need to create local people living with HIV groups was central, since after testing there were no treatment resources available. The hope was that people in these groups would help each other. In conversation at one well established international NGO that specialized in agricultural extension work, the country director said that '… it was important to diversify what we do as funding for our main work was not increasing. This year we have done a lot of VCT by using the access we had in the rural areas'. He went on to say that, 'next year it is not clear as funding focus seems to change may be we focus on orphan situation, we are not sure whether we will carry on with VCT work'. When asked where he saw the added value in this work, his response was 'we [have] worked in the country long time and we know many communities, so this helps us to do VCT roll out. We cannot stay too long in each location as we need to cover many communities [so] we encourage people once we give them their results to get together with others who were tested to support each other'.

I observed a similar situation at about the same time in a capital city in southern Africa where I found that there was an active people living with HIV group. Talking to the members was interesting, especially when they explained their work was very hard. As one member put it, 'we are doing advocacy work to overcome stigma and raise awareness to get people be tested but we need help. We have no resources to help us in between when we go to meet internationals'. I was told that 'life is hard, particularly now we know our status and we try to support each other without medicine or other support what can we do'. As a local group, they had formed around the health clinic members had been tested at and once they had formed they were asked to go and talk in schools and work places, and to be open publically about their status as part of a broader policy initiative to share information to change behaviour. Yet, the group did not seem to have any leverage with policy makers. This was a time when treatment was not broadly available and only a limited number of treatment facilities existed in Sub-Saharan Africa. One of the participants in the discussion said that 'we are told that there will be some treatment but who will get it, they will have a small amount. Who will decide who gets it'? Other members talked about the difficulties they had as individuals outside the group. In a way they were a civil society initiative, probably a project supported by an international policy actor, and as such they were part of the Global AIDS framework. However, they did not have the capacity to change or influence the policies targeting them – either within the AIDS policy field or beyond.

These reflections from Sub-Saharan Africa are about the creation and operation of local groups. They also reveal how civil society practice is often coordinated as a part of a larger global policy framework. But the processes of coordination lead to co-option when there are resource imbalances resulting in limited agency development and only then within the Global AIDS framework. This can be seen in the way many groups have had to change what they do to remain relevant within global resource relations as Global AIDS priorities change. Whatever funding was available for intervention priorities at a given time motivates local groups to deliver on these priorities. Here, I recognize that the relationship between local and global actors is dynamic, and that local actors can assert their agency by valorising their HIV commitment and status according to the degree to which AIDS is seen as a public health priority at a specific time and place. However, while fast-growing AIDS-related NGOs and community groups in many local spaces have been trying to address local problems, they have also been becoming more responsive to and constrained within Global AIDS and the priorities it sets.

4.5 Categories of Co-option and Solidarity

The process of diffusion of policy categories can also be seen as co-option into the broader global AIDS policy framework. The idea of co-option, here, is about how the use of particular categories makes certain people more relevant to the Global AIDS concerns that guide action in relation to them. By creating communities of policy, not only with respect to NGOs but also targeted groups, people's ways of acting are framed. The life of the concept of MSM is interesting in this regard is interesting. From the moment the term first emerged as a policy category to target people's behaviours rather than identities (Seckinelgin 2009b) to the formation of The Global Forum on MSM and HIV (MSMGF) in 2006, we can witness a dynamic process – from the term being used first a tool to target socially marginalized people, to becoming a near-identity, to influencing the behaviours of others as a global signifier across different country contexts. At a workshop in India in the second half of the 2000s, which I co-organized on the theme of *Marginalized Sexualities and AIDS,* one female Indian participant from Calcutta confronted many of the other participants when she said

> … before AIDS, we had solidarity among many different sexuality groups to organize and claim our rights. Now because all [the] funds on AIDS are targeting [towards] MSM, there is no solidarity. If you cannot fit within these target groups, you lose your voice as activism is more organized around AIDS to benefit from funding than actual issues on sexuality. We, as lesbians, disappeared from public debate.

Many of the other participants from within India admitted that she was correct and that the only way to obtain funding for their sexuality-related work was by rebranding their sexuality activism as AIDS activism under a public health concern. This exchange, among many other similar exchanges in India and in Africa, highlights the ways in which the global AIDS-policy categories have interacted with already existing civil society activism. It also shows how local actors appropriate international support and funding and convert these into resources that they redeploy for their own purposes. In such processes we can observe a number of dynamics. First, success in achieving a funding goal rests with belonging to a network – the Global AIDS network – and having credibility within it. Second, within this networked activity there is a power dependence, as one set of actors changes their outlook to become part of the resourcing relationship. Third, such actions lead to imbalanced interdependencies within the Global AIDS system – local actors' survival rests on the continuity and integrity of this relationship, while the credibility of the claims of the Global AIDS system requires showing diffused but working relations with a variety of community activists.

At the same meeting in India, a well-known activist who I had met a year earlier during my research at his own NGO which dealt with particular group of men and their HIV-related issues in Mumbai, argued that independent of all of the identity differences among sexuality groups 'we are all MSM now'. I was very surprised at this, given the strong stance he had taken a year before against the kind of homogenization of different groups. His MSM argument generated heated debate led by a leading local hijra activist who argued that 'I am not, we are not, MSM – we are hijra we are culturally accepted within our [own] culture. The MSM approach is not helpful to deal with our problems around economic and social exclusion'. The first activist responded, 'that might be true, but the MSM category is the way to go as many international organizations are focusing on the issue through this category, and there is no way to resist to it if you want to be part of the process'. This was a dramatic confrontation which lasted quite some time. The first activist's position was based on a realistic assessment of funding allocations targeting a particular category of people. The shift here was a practical one: to be able to have access to resources and be heard by global actors such as UNAIDS, he had had to change his position. The position of the hijra activist was also important. She was making a rights-based claim for differentiated needs by resisting the attempt to reduce these claims to a policy category that targeted deliverable technical interventions. This interchange offers an example of how the international and the local interact to transformative effect, and how global categories globalize particular activists as they begin to use that particular language. Their voices come to represent those who are targeted by particular policy categories as they are incorporated into the Global AIDS process.

This subtle co-option by categories can take a more direct form, for example, when many successful local civil society activists and leaders end up working for international organizations including international NGOs on AIDS. Here I am talking about a dynamic relationship based on the movement of ideas and people between various spaces of activism. At a local level, the space for activism is framed within a national socio-political context, while at the global level activism takes place within a different logic. The process of movement takes place not only between local NGOs and international organizations such as UNAIDS, but between international umbrella/network organizations for civil society groups and these same international organizations.

Throughout such transformations two important processes can be observed. In the case of MSM, it is possible to see how MSM has become a code, a category, through which to address gay men's needs in resource-poor settings. It has brought forth new resources through the use of a public health category, in some cases in countries where homosexual behaviour between men is illegal. Beyond this, however, there is a resonance between the category and civil society activism. While numerous community groups have been formed in relation to the MSM category, there has also been the emergence of network organizations such as MSMGF and African Men for Sexual Health and Rights (AMSHeR), creating platforms through which sexual minority men's needs can be located within a rights framework. In the organisation's webpages, MSMGF's is described as being

> founded in 2006 at the International AIDS Conference in Toronto by activists from around the world concerned about the silence surrounding HIV among men who have sex with men, including gay and bisexual men. MSMGF was born out of an urgent need to act. (MSMGF 2016a)

This narrative locates the need for MSMGF within the lack of substantive policy discussion on MSM and related sexuality issues within the already well established Global AIDS community. AMSHeR's creation also derives from within this same context.[18] In a sense, therefore, their emergence posed an internal challenge to the Global AIDS approach. While the challenge was well timed, it has also consolidated the process of turning MSM into an identity, which could be claimed in order to have access to resources and rights. It is also clear that through this dynamic, for instance, MSMGF has been able to engage legitimately with a range of Global AIDS actors and thereby stake a representational claim to speak on behalf of others.[19] AMSHeR also shares this outlook. As a network organization of 18 separate organizations from across Africa, it acts as the facilitator for local group development and activism. These network organizations work and 'function as a management knot' (Pape 2014:215). They are also highly professionalized. While they run their own research programs in coordination with other global AIDS actors, they also manage the work and participation of local constituent civil society groups.

[18] The idea for its creation emerged in discussion between HIV and human rights activists after the International Conference on AIDS and STIs in Africa (ICASA) in Abuja in 2005. Discussion later intensified at the 2008 International AIDS Conference in Mexico City, leading to AMSHeR's formal establishment in 2009 (AMSHER 2016). The organization's pre-conference in Addis Ababa in 2011 at the 16th ICASA meeting was disrupted by conservative anti-homosexuality groups and their venue moved to a UN provided space from the originally planned venue at the Jupiter International hotel (ILGA 2011and mambaonline 2011).

[19] A review of a number of their annual reports shows that gradually MSMGF has become one of the key civil society groups participating in global policy debates on HIV.

Thus, they act as nodes through which they diffuse particular policy priorities, policy frames and tools for action.[20]

In addition to organizing its own research and policy engagements through its Africa-wide pre-conference workshops on MSM at International Conferences on AIDS and STIs in Africa [ICASA], AMSHeR has brought African activists together to build 'home grown strategies to address local issues' (AMSHER 2016). I observed this in presentations delivered persuasively by AMSHER activists in number of public AIDS-related events where global experts' help was questioned for its appropriateness in line with African socio-political realities. Then, at a pre-conference MSM workshop organized by AMSHeR in December 2013 at the ICASA conference in Cape Town. I observed a change of dynamics. At this meeting there were about 160–170 people broadly comprised of activists and NGO representatives from across Africa together with people from different Global AIDS organizations. The event was sponsored by a number of international organizations and international civil society groups which include MSMGF, HiVOS-people unlimited, the International HIV/AIDS Alliance, the Ford Foundation, the Global Fund to Fight AIDS, Tuberculosis and Malaria, UNAIDS, UNDP and UNFPA and others. The presence of so many top level organisations in the same meeting highlights the close relationship between these organizations. The meeting was opened by Michel Sidibé, the Executive Director of UNAIDS, whose speech on stigma, homophobia and AIDS proved important. He implicitly acknowledged the silence on these issues and the way that change was taking place on these issues within UNAIDS. He argued that change had to happen and argued that 'stigma is not only in the courtroom but in the home too'. After reminding people of the problems faced at the IACASA in Addis Ababa in 2011 and the work developed by AMSHeR since then on violence and human rights, he talked about how MSM were especially vulnerable to HIV by presenting prevalence rates from a number of African countries and the problem, for instance, of poor access to lubricants. He said, 'we cannot ignore the growing epidemic' and that UNAIDS is working on various issues that include rights affirming intervention models and renewed activism'. He acknowledged that doing so could be tricky in countries where same-sex relations were criminalized but pointed to the importance of the visibility of local efforts. Talking of such situations, he said that 'I know UNAIDS does not always support you or take your position… I sent a letter [to country staff] that they need to support you (MSM) at the country level and… (with respect to) HIV and health needs. In many cases my advice is not amplified. I want that to change. If they [UNAIDS local staff] cannot [do this], I say the risk they are taking is they are not representing me. Someone told me that [if they did] they could become a *persona non grata*. I said, I will promote you if you are kicked out of a country because you fight for [people's] rights and [against] discrimination. You deserve to be promoted'. Then, he added. 'We want to be part of your journey for justice'.

[20]This process could also be seen in the particular role played by NGOs for 'global social governance' to help regulate and redistribute towards achieving particular global policy outcomes (Kruse and Martens 2015:184–87).

This was a remarkable statement, which also highlighted a problem in the Global AIDS framework being managed by UNAIDS. We can think about it further through linkage to following observation 'UNAIDS estimates HIV prevalence to be 17.9 % among MSM in SSA [Sub-Saharan Africa]. Yet there are limited epidemiological data for MSM or KPs [key populations] in general in this region' (Wolf et al. 2013: 1). This lack of data suggests that UNAIDS has found it politically difficult to engage in this debate since its inception.[21] Sidibé's speech here was not only an attempt to revive the relationship between UNAIDS and the activist community, but also about showing that UNAIDS agreed with the need to comprehensively support MSM activism as a part of the Global AIDS response. Considering there were representatives from many funders and donors present, the speech was also about stressing the role of UNAIDS and its will to engage dynamically in the debate. Arguably Sidibé's intervention is an instrumental one to emphasize the importance of UNAIDS.[22] The tone of the messages – both from Sidibé and from the next speaker – was one of determination and readiness for confrontation. He then introduced the former Vice-President of Uganda, Specioza Wandira Kazibwe, who had been appointed by Ban-Ki Moon as a United Nations Special envoy on AIDS in Africa. She began her speech by saying that as 'the mother of twins … in our culture I can say anything' – speak truth to the power – and that she has never been deterred from controversy. In talking against homophobia, she talked about demystifying 'sexual organs…sexual organ where you put it or where you are not suppose to put it…it is in your head if it is not in your head it does not matter where you put it if you enjoy it'.

While plenary sessions at this meeting were framed in a capacity building modality, other panel sessions were more about hearing from experiences. One of the main themes at the event concerned the violation of MSM/LGBTI human rights and how to address this. It was in this debate that I observed the shift in the language used by number of leading activists. The strategic use of the law was presented as an important tool for dealing with human rights issues. One important aspect of this concerned the use of already existing African human rights mechanisms, some of which were linked with the African Charter on Human and People's Rights, and the protection it offers against violence. However, a number of people suggested that this particular strategy would not work at home because they did not have lawyers who were willing to engage in this process. One response to this was that support could be provided through lawyers' networks in other countries, including South Africa. A question was put to the legal panel about whether such an approach might lead to further violence and criminalization. Before the panel could answer, one of

[21] This situation is to a degree context dependent, since MSM issues have been addressed through UNAIDS work in other parts of the world. Conducting research in Myanmar in the autumn of 2014, it was clear UNAIDS in that country (where homosexual relations between men are also illegal) was developing a strategy to conduct a major survey among MSM. While this was important, the stigma and hard-to-reach nature of MSM in Myanmar present important challenges in that context.

[22] It was not, however, clear how far Sidibé is able provide support for grounded engagement with the causes of the problem.

the lead activists organizing the event responded from the floor by saying that 'you cannot make an omelet without breaking eggs' to indicate the inevitably of negative outcomes in the short term. I was very surprised, as the same activist had some months earlier in a different meeting challenged a major international NGO that had proposed the idea that he was now supporting – namely, the strategic use of legal means in Africa. At that time he had said 'Don't do it, we know how to handle our own socio-political relations and how act within those, you don't'. When I asked the director of another INGO sitting next to me about this, she did not express any surprise. She explained, 'He is a good politician and knowing all the donors and INGOs in the room', he is 'showing that he is on the same page as many of these actors'. Her comments offered an evaluation the activist's performance of his brokerage role. He recognized the multiple realities associated with his position through actions which signaled the need to play a different role in the presence of power (Long 1992).

The strategic use of the law discussed in these events was however based on abstracting the modality from its context. The arguments presented ignored when and where such an approach might be useful. In the absence of such scrutiny, it is perhaps premature to expect litigation on its own to initiate major change in a given society.[23] The approach also revealed some of the limitations of the didactic nature of the event, limitations which could also be observed in a number of panel sessions. When a presenter provided information that did not fit the overall narrative, the issues raised did not get much of a hearing. For instance, one representative of a local organization from western Africa talked about the way in which in his country access to HIV-related resources were broadly fine and how many MSM had access to them, even though the law criminalized same-sex relations. He also added that the law has rarely been used, saying, 'You hear about rape or violence [but] you don't hear about homosexuality when two men are arrested'. He then talked about the existence of a generalized social homophobia in the country but added that given general social attitudes people in their everyday lives are not generally homophobic. Only when the topic comes up does homophobia rise, being 'reinforced by media and religious groups who use [the] media to advertise'. His presentation provided a rather nuanced analysis of how to think about overcoming homophobia in his context. But these nuances were not picked up by the audience, with the chair of the panel reflecting on what they might suggest for the more generalized promotion of the intervention strategies that we were hearing about at the workshop.

Rather than reflecting on these issues contextually, a representative of the Global Fund to Fight AIDS, Tuberculosis and Malaria provided the generic suggestion that 'MSM groups should use this new opportunity [Country Dialogues] to get funding or engage their governments on legal reform, legal architecture, and HR architecture

[23] One of the origins of this law-based tool lies in the civil rights movements in the USA where law, broader citizenship rights and other socio-political tools contributed to the important outcomes such as the desegregation of education through the courts (see Alexander 2012). Similar success can be seen with respect to outcomes from the work of The AIDS Law Project in South Africa (Mbali 2013; Hart 2015).

and how they could be changed'. She did this in an effort to help, but it was clear that she did not consider the different socio-political context within which activism occurred and which we had been hearing about throughout the day. Arguably, civil society groups were given a new tool – strategic litigation – to work with in the form of the strategic use of the law, but this tool did not engage with the sources of stigma that ground legal thinking and legal action in many countries. What was clear from many of the presentations was that they were describing projects to show the dynamism of the MSM communities, and to show success in efforts to reinforce the Global AIDS message of hope in the face of adversity. The underlying theme was one of progressively achieving positive outcomes through the use of the means that are promoted as relevant by regional and international experts and funded broadly by the Global AIDS collective.

International conferences and workshops provide opportunities to exchange ideas and get to know about new policy tools. They function as the centre of the 'chain of communication and interpretation' required for the policy transfers facilitated by Global AIDS actors (McCabe 2007: 207). The transfer process is also underwritten by the Global AIDS solidarity performed on such occasions. While the major International AIDS Society conferences now take place every 2 years, there are regional conferences such as ICASA between these larger events. These biennial conferences attract many thousands of people. Their organization is a complex process, as different elements and constituents have to be accommodated within the conference programme. At these events, the spirit of civil society activism is maintained at least formally, since the IAS itself is a civil society organization. The conferences highlight the contribution of a range of actors involved in Global AIDS. While bodies such as UNAIDS, WHO, the World Bank and The Global Fund to Fight AIDS, Tuberculosis and Malaria, participate in the proceedings, the events give the impression that they are open spaces at which a variety of participants have a platform. These are also about the trust building process, where trust is about the 'willingness to take some risks in relation to other individuals on the expectation that the others will reciprocate' (Walker and Ostrom 2005: 382). There is a sense in which international organizations take a back step from the centre stage, which is occupied by the scientists and civil society activists in line with the GIPA principles. However, much of this trust building is also illusionary. Most of the international civil society groups and activists participating in these events do so through funding provided by the international organizations and international NGOs that are part of Global AIDS. These organisations use funds to bring local partners from different countries to showcase particular projects. In this way, the Global AIDS system showcases what it has achieved by reiterating the importance of participants keeping the system supported, by remaining within the horizons set by these showcasing events.

As Shilts (1988) has observed, in recent years these conferences have become much institutionalized events where science, activism, policy actors and business interact. However, these interactions are strictly regulated. While the participation of HIV positive people and members of civil society is central, their contributions are usually located in different parts of the conference programme from the scientific panels where new medical discoveries are discussed. While there may be civil society panels where NGOs present their work, these are not the main focus of the conference or the centre of debate. It is hard not to think that many of these side-events are organized to fulfil the IAS's civil society role and to give token voice to activists and local groups rather than allow them to have influence over the main substance of debate. These panels are often occasions with much lower attendance than the panels at which high profile scientists and representatives from the main international organizations speak. The representational rationale motivating this process maintains a segregated outlook.

Certainly, those attending the conferences can observe the participation of numerous civil society groups, policy actors and the private sector form across the globe. Private sector actors and foundations organize satellite meetings before the main conference programme to promote their own products or programmes. There are also designated exhibition areas with stands to promote new technological and medical products. Typically, what is called the Global Village (a specialist conference area) provides a space where civil society groups and activists can meet for the duration of the conference. Here, smaller NGOs and groups, as exhibitors, promote their work; there is also a discussion programme with panels organized by different groups. It is within the Global Village that some of the most critical discussions. Separation between the main conference and the Global Village highlights the way in which civil society is included. It is given space but is not entirely integrated into the main debate.

One example of the rather tense relationship between science and activism took place at the AIDS 2012 conference in Washington DC. At a press conference at the start of the meeting, chaired by the then executive director of IAS, the conference programme chairs, the executive director of UNAIDS and others, a demonstration interrupted the panel. Standing up with the slogan *No Drug Users, No Sex-Workers*, and moving down to the stage and walking back up to exit the venue, activists disrupted the beginning of the press conference. The chair of the panel announced 'For those of you who did not know there is a [US] travel ban for sex workers and drug users, and now you know. And thank you for that' (AIDS 2012a). The reaction of the chair and the panel members was one of complicity. They gave space to civil society activists to do what they wanted for few minutes before getting on with the more serious work. Their actions purported to show that all are part of civil society, while guiding and limiting the impact of the demonstration.

Policy makers from governments and international organizations are invited to address the conference and indeed there is a sense of giving an account of their activities to the community. One of the politicians who sent a video recorded speech to the AIDS 2014 Washington conference was the then US Secretary of State Hillary Clinton, who delivered a passionate and supportive message welcoming everyone to Washington DC (AIDS 2012b). Some of these plenary sessions have up to 5000 people in the audience. Many activists and scientists were also asked to give keynote addresses to the conference, either to talk about their experiences as activists and the importance of the continuing fight against AIDS, or to talk as scientists about promising new breakthroughs in dealing with HIV. Through this process, HIV positive people and civil society participation show why 'all of us' in the form of the Global AIDS community still needs to fight against AIDS and why the science presented matters. While the conferences still present some science, they also have become a civil society space which allows for the idea of Global AIDS solidarity to be performed, and reiterated. This reiteration is often accomplished by focusing each conference on a civil society concern to significantly 'improve rates of cooperation' between activists and the Global AIDS system (see Walker and Ostrom 2009:103). This tactic allows for a constant rejuvenating of the idea of the AIDS movement and global AIDS community, while showing the outside world the movement is still strong and remains an important political actor.

4.6 Conclusion

In this chapter, I have tried to trace some of the key transformations in the civil society response to HIV and the way in which this has become a part of the Global AIDS system. The increased numbers of NGOs engaged in AIDS-related activity serves to demonstrate the existence, vibrancy and the nature of the global AIDS movement, providing legitimacy for the view that the epidemic requires an emergency response. The assumption here is that the civil society activism that was so successful in the earlier stages of HIV epidemic during the 1980s and early 1990s can also be generated elsewhere. However, in contrast to the past, civil society organisations in resource-poor settings nowadays tend to formed as policy communities guided not so much by local interests as by Global AIDS imperatives (Seckinelgin 2012b). This partaking in Global AIDS has turned many local groups into brokers and 'those who breathe life into transnational projects, mediating between different constituencies to make those projects possible' (Thoreson 2014: 11). While arguably this may provide some groups with political leverage in their own countries, the brokerage role has not turned them into agents of political change independent of the larger Global AIDS collective. Instead, a Global AIDS framework has come to define the pathway to dealing with the problem, largely limiting the agency of civil society groups to the management and implementation of local projects on behalf of the international AIDS movement. To this day, many NGO interventions remain at best pilot projects that lack funding or socio-political support within the context in which they have been implemented. It remains uncertain whether these activities will in the end create or lead to sustainable change. It is also questionable whether the civil society infrastructure that has emerged and developed in response to Global AIDS and its emergency thinking can survive on its own.

Chapter 5
Global AIDS and the Politics of Knowledge

In this chapter, I want to examine how the policy priorities of Global AIDS have informed the nature of knowledge developed in this field. I want also to suggest that how knowledge on HIV has developed highlights some important features of the Global AIDS system. From early beginnings in the 1980s, our knowledge of HIV has expanded rapidly. Many new policies to address HIV have been developed on the back of this growing knowledge base. However, while this expansion has been important, it conceals a central weakness. This weakness stems from the way in which specifically bio-medical knowledge has been deployed for policy development processes within the Global AIDS framework. In particular, while scientific knowledge of HIV has grown, it has done so in the absence of experience-based local knowledge. This sets limits on how applicable biomedically informed policy can be, and highlights the challenges of implementing generic public health interventions in particular local settings.

This weakness also highlights another major problem in relation to the future of such policies. As discussed in the introduction, the future of HIV in many contexts is about the sustainability of existing policy interventions and sustainable change over time to address people's particular needs as they evolve. Due to changes in international aid flows in the last few decades, one of the priorities of the Global AIDS system has been to encourage local governments to take over many responsibility for many of the interventions initiated and supported by international funding. The critical issue here is one of localising knowledge production processes so that these can support policy development over time. However, the domain of knowledge production remains firmly located in resource-rich settings. This dominates the way in which knowledge is translated into policy priorities as part of the Global AIDS approach. Research investment remains located mostly in resource-rich settings to expedite policy development for dealing with a health 'emergency', as Global AIDS defines the problem. While numerous bio-medical trials have been conducted in developing countries and local scientists participate in these processes, it is not clear how much research capacity has been built in resource-poor settings for sustained engagement with the policy process (Epstein 2007).

H. Seckinelgin, *The Politics of Global AIDS*, Social Aspects of HIV 3,
DOI 10.1007/978-3-319-46013-0_5

For many scholars who have participated in these discussions, the debate is often about the dominance of bio-medical knowledge claims over the knowledge produced by the social sciences. For instance a wide-ranging review of social science knowledge production and its contributions to the global AIDS debate commissioned by the International AIDS Society argued that '[a]ppreciation of the significant role that the social and political sciences have played in HIV prevention, treatment and care has declined as the focus on treatment and biomedical prevention technologies has grown stronger' (Kippax and Holt 2009: 3). In this review, Susan Kippax and Martin Holt consider the limited opportunities for the social sciences to publish in high profile AIDS-related journals, highlighting the dominance given to bio-medical research instead. It is hard not to agree with their observations. Kippax and Holt argue that 'many papers ostensibly published on social or political science [are] primarily concerned with HIV interventions; this was the case across all of the journals we reviewed. There were considerably fewer publications on the social and political "drivers" of HIV epidemics' (2009:3). This is an important observation in that it suggests that 'the readership of specialist HIV journals is unlikely to be well informed about current developments in social and political research' (2009:3). Their account also draws attention to the particular knowledge production system that gives value to research according to categories that are seen as relevant to the policy needs of the Global AIDS system. It points to the existence of a hierarchy of knowledge based on the perceived relevance of different kinds of research for dealing with HIV and AIDS in general: moving from medical science to implementation. Here, the question is about how research from within the social and political sciences may be relevant to HIV policy implementation needs.

In focusing in on this, I want to look at the issue not merely from the binary positioning of the bio-medical versus the social sciences. The above observed change in how social sciences are considered within the field is due not only to advance in scientific and medical technologies, but also to a shared orientation between biomedicine's approach to the disease and the way in which international organizations in their global health concerns have become interested in population-level policy interventions. It is this shared orientation that underwrites the Global AIDS approach. As explained earlier, this biomedically informed global policy stance arose from the juncture of 1980s activism on the one hand (Callon et al. 84: 2009) and policy expediency to locate resources at a time of emergency in the 1990s, on the other. This conjuncture enabled 'scientists [to] play their role as problem solvers' (Hisschemoller et al. 2001:447–9). This process also functioned to set out and define the nature of the problem, policy priorities and target groups that would need help from within the Global AIDS framework. As Margaret Lock and Vinh-Kim Nguyen argue, 'biological technologies have the prime function of enabling humans to act on the world and its people' (2010:20). It is this enabling possibility which links biomedical thinking closely to the global gaze of the international actors who are looking at HIV-related populations.

The assumption that is made here is about the way in which biomedical technologies are considered to produce effects that are 'essentially uniform whenever they are put into operation' (Lock and Nguyen 2010:6). This assumption only becomes possible when there is an 'excessive desire to regard any sick body as equivalent to any other sick body' (Callon et al. 2009:85). The desire to do good is embedded in common medical science assumptions that allow human body to considered as 'readily ...standardizable by means of systematic assessments, bringing about a further assumption that the material make-up of the body is, for all intents and purposes universal' (Lock and Nguyen 2010:20). Lock and Nguyen point out that this perspective is closely related to the social goal of clinical biomedicine, which 'is ...one of pinpointing internal bodily truths' (2010:42), and also to the claim that 'biomedicine, because it is grounded in science, has a special status based on objectivity and standardization independent of society and culture' (Lock and Nguyen 2010: 53).

These are informative assumptions for understanding why a biomedical approach has underwritten the Global AIDS system with its focus on dealing with *disease* and not on people *living with the HIV* in particular socio-cultural settings. Biomedical assumptions and the policy directions following from these assumptions enables a focusing on generic bodies that have HIV. This in turn helps global policy thinking to formulate policies targeting HIV in these bodies, both to provide treatment and to stop HIV being transmitted to others. The way in which AIDS becomes a global concern on the basis of its biomedical construction also helps policy makers maintain Global AIDS as a framework.[1] Biomedical knowledge and the possibility of turning this knowledge into technologies to target HIV generically across often very different settings allow international policy makers to think globally, because they can then cross boundaries without engaging with socio-cultural and political issues – just so long as they are dealing with 'AIDS'.

This move from biomedical knowledge to policy-relevant biotechnologies that can help policy actors address the disease also concerns cost-effectiveness. The need to localise generic biomedical knowledge to enabling thinking about the disease in particular bodies in particular contexts, presents generates a major funding problem. In consequence, biotechnical intervention abstracts the disease from its setting, constructing it as a generic biomedical condition that can be dealt with independent of the way in which people experience it. As Lock and Nguyen argue, 'once technological interventions become the keys to diagnosis and to care the inevitable changes result as to what counts as valid knowledge about the body, the doctor – patient relationship, and indeed, the relationship among the body, culture and society' (2010:20). This gives rise to a larger process of medicalization which seeks to incorporate within its boundaries all other forms of knowledge production, including those of the social sciences. By setting the perceived validity of biomedical assumptions and modalities as the measure against which Global AIDS policy relevant knowledge must be judged, this process builds on the 'ideational capacities of

[1] I would like to emphasize here that this discussion is about the way in which the perceptions of biomedicine that exist within the policy world inform the way in which key actors within this world use these perspectives to engage with biomedical knowledge. It is often the case that at the level of clinical engagement many, medically trained professionals think about what they are doing in relation the individual circumstances an individual faces.

actors who possess specialized knowledge as a form of "epistemic" authority that derives from their status within a particular community of experts' (Broome and Seabrooke 2015: 958), in this case from within the Global AIDS framework itself. Given also that most of the actors with this presumed ideational capacity are located in resource-rich settings, the possibility of addressing policy needs in resource-poor settings becomes inherently linked to power relationships within the Global AIDS system.

I argue, therefore, that the issue medicalization is less about the fact that AIDS is framed in this manner than about the way in which biomedical knowledge comes to be deployed by key actors to develop and manage the Global AIDS approach in general (see Clarke et al. 2010; Seckinelgin 2008). This engagement with biomedicine from within the Global AIDS policy interest seeks to evaluate all knowledge related to HIV from within this lens. As a result, the approach deploys the model of biomedical thinking and its assumptions, described above, as *the* required model of knowledge on Global AIDS in general. Using this lens, enduring and complex social-science-related questions are reduced to problems to be tackled through 'intervention' and eradicated.[2] For example, poverty, gender inequalities, stigma and even homophobia become issues to be targeted through silver bullet interventions directed towards 'key populations', without engaging with the socio-cultural, political and economic conditions that underpin these concerns. This diagnostic approach reduces the specificities created by these conditions to HIV-related social facts/problems that we need to target. Arguably, the human rights approach to HIV offers some counter to this but, as discussed in the previous chapter, despite its rhetorical appeal such an approach has had limited impact. Even when it made access to antiretroviral treatment a global human rights issue, this has not moved beyond focusing on getting pills to people, and not on what happens to them as they have the treatment over time.

5.1 Rethinking Debate on Biomedicine Versus the Social Sciences

I am arguing here that the knowledge practices of international HIV discourse reflect the particular ways in which the Global AIDS system has developed. As Charles Taylor, quoted in Descombes (2014: 299) puts it,

> … the meanings and norms implicit in these practices are not just in the minds of the actors but are out there in the practices themselves, practices which cannot be conceived as set of individual actions, but which are essentially modes of social relation, of mutual action

Particular generic biomedical knowledge is considered central to international AIDS policy because of the social relations between the key actors involved

[2] See, for instance, Knutsson (2016) considers what it means to achieve AIDS-related positive outcomes in the politically constrained environment of Rwanda.

including the international organizations and the international NGOs that take part in the reproduction of Global AIDS. From the early emergence of AIDS activism, the movement found 'a place in the public domain in as much as the associations involved bringing together many doctors, intellectuals, and scientists' (Callon et al. 2009: 84). This framing has positioned much policy thinking by bringing together biomedical imperatives, scientific expertise and the need to reach out globally as a way of thinking and acting. Such a perspective grounds the Global AIDS system and its institutions, framing, incentivising and supporting particular ways of knowing and acting as a 'conceptual system'(Descombes 2014: 301)

I have argued that focusing on the dichotomy between biomedicine and social sciences is not very helpful since it ignores this broader foundational constraint and ends up being a discussion of what is to be included in the Global AIDS response. This too readily turns to the question of how the social sciences to be are evaluated in terms of their relevance to Global AIDS. The possibility of their inclusion becomes limited to how far different knowledge production practices can be rendered comprehensible within the global AIDS framework as a conceptual system. Thus, the social sciences only become relevant within the Global AIDS system as useful tools for and limited by implementation science. This view in turn is legitimated by the need for mutual action in *solidarity* to tackle a common technical objective. Such an approach frames and establishes a division of labour between different knowledge practices according to their perceived utility. At the same time, however, biomedical knowledge remains unchallenged as the over-arching epistemological and conceptual system, unquestioned in its centrality to Global AIDS relevance.

Focusing in on the definition of implementation science is instructive here. According to the definition provided by the Fogarty International Centre of US National Institutes of Health (2016:1), implementation science is

> ....the study of methods to promote the integration of research findings and evidence into healthcare policy and practice. It seeks to understand the behavior of healthcare professionals and other stakeholders as a key variable in the sustainable uptake, adoption, and implementation of evidence-based interventions
>
> It aims
>
> ... to investigate and address major bottlenecks (e.g. social, behavioral, economic, management) that impede effective implementation, test new approaches to improve health programming, as well as determine a causal relationship between the intervention and its impact.

This instrumental approach to the use of the social sciences selects and limits the kind of research that is perceived as useful to the Global AIDS policy needs. It does this by directly raising the question of relevance, evaluating this according to biomedical understandings and utility. Here, notions of implementation limit social science interest to policy delivery, that is to 'translating policy into action' (Barrett 2004: 251). Policy in its broadest sense is quickly reduced to 'policy content' as determined by bio-medicine and implementation concerns – a technical matter beyond the scientific content associated with it. Policy content then becomes a truth claim about HIV and AIDS in general.

Because of this, the drive to be included in Global AIDS debate places many social scientists in the position of servicing already established priorities and needs, rather than considering HIV from their own position. This leads to a filtering of the kind of social research that is considered relevant. Kippax and Holt note this when they describe how

> … social science is often reduced to behavioral research by funding bodies and by conference organizers, including the International AIDS Society…[this] overemphasis on behavioral research displays a poor understanding of the range of social science research approaches and preference for individualized research paradigms (2009:54).

5.2 The Diffusion of Knowledge and Its Limits

I have already discussed the biennial World AIDS Conferences organised by the International AIDS Society (IAS) as key settings for civil society action. I want now to examine these conference spaces as training grounds or fields in which particular kinds of knowledge are diffused and the Global AIDS system is reproduced. As training grounds, different actors are socialized through IAS conferences into the Global AIDS system. Together with regional meetings organised by IAS and its partners, they provide a 'structured contact targeted at the transfer of rules' and ways of thinking about AIDS (Freyburg 2015: 63). The mechanism of conferences 'aims to foster emulation and a shared policy language among a community of actors' (Broome and Seabrooke 2015: 956). Furthermore, through conference socialization particular ways of thinking on AIDS may be taught 'to a community of actors that change how they conceive of their collective identity and interest' (Chekel 2005: 804). Via this process of creating shared knowledge and skills, the ability to participate properly in Global AIDS is developed as 'policy networks are ever more centred on those who can demonstrate that their professional skills and professionalization are transnational rather than remaining in national systems' (Seabrooke 2014:1).

In particular AIDS conferences provide venues for different actors to 'participate' in Global AIDS debate through 'practice-based forms of learning and direct engagement in deliberation over policy problems' (Broome and Seabrooke 2015: 958; Freyburg 2015). Practice-based forms of learning are especially evident in the way in which common problems and common policy solutions are identified. By discussing these, 'a shared vocabulary' in the form of the language of Global AIDS (or Global AIDS speak) is communicated and diffused (Broome and Seabrooke 2015: 966). In the end, participants become aware of the 'state-of-the art' policy thinking, priorities and international 'best-practices'. They acquire a common language that they then use in engaging with these issues once they return back to their everyday settings (Broome and Seabrooke 2015: 963). Back at home, they then become AIDS 'policy entrepreneurs' linking those settings with the Global AIDS system (Kingdon 1995; Finnemore and Sikkink 1998).[3]

Given the way in which biomedical knowledge grounds knowledge production and limits relevance claims, AIDS conferences as civil society spaces function within a particular power relationship. They bring together two key groups of people: those who produce the perceived relevant knowledge that centrally frames AIDS and those who are learning about this knowledge and its possible uses. Here Leonard Seabrooke's (2014) concept of 'epistemic arbitrage' is relevant. This concept is about understanding 'how particular professionals are able to exploit differences in professional knowledge pools for strategic advantage by positioning particular forms of knowledge as the most appropriate to deal with particular problems' (2014:2). The possibility of particular professionals claiming to have more knowledge, and the exploitation of differences in knowledge with respect to the Global AIDS case, rests on the relationship established between biomedical scientists and the international policy actors who provide direction for the required knowledge. From this point of view, conferences offer a process through which biomedical scientists not only reproduce their centrality to the future of AIDS and their view on life as that most relevant to dealing with AIDS globally, but they also reproduce the boundaries governing others' participation in AIDS debates through this process. And, as discussed above, the idea of looking at knowledge from an implementation science perspective is one of these boundary-making processes.

But, how does this become possible? Seabrooke argues that when this process is 'successful, those engaging in epistemic arbitrage become epistemic "arbiters" who decide how to address the transnational problems and who can address them' (2014:2). This allows professionals to carve out an imbalanced power position, which is often reproduced within the conference processes. The key issue here is about the way in which certain groups get to establish themselves as more 'expert' than others, and reproduce their position within what is claimed to be the wider AIDS movement at the conferences. Seabrooke points out that epistemological arbitrage 'is based on a relationship in which a professional is identified as "knowing well" rather than simply having a stock of information (2014:3). A key issue here is the cyclical relationship that establishes who knows well, from the way in which AIDS is framed as a medical problem, which makes biomedicine central to solving the problem and then leads to the establishment of particular knowledge claims as relevant. Once the boundaries of the latter have been set as relevant, this requires that biomedical scientists lead the debate. In this way, knowing well is intimately linked to biomedical knowledge that has global reach. This also reduces the importance of other ways of knowing well, such as through experience-based knowledge claims. Significantly, policy demands within the Global AIDS system make the

---

[3] This learning process allows many people over time to move professionally between various organizational settings within the Global AIDS system. As I discussed in earlier chapters, some of the key ways of doing Global AIDS work are related to activists' movement from resource-rich settings into international organizations. Similarly, many AIDS workers from resource-poor settings can become global activists by working for or alongside international organizations.

generalizability of knowledge for policy purposes a condition of knowing well. What Seabrooke recognises here is not about whether in some objective sense biomedical scientists have the knowledge to be justified in their claim to know well or not. His useful insight lies in the fact that epistemic arbitrage is 'based on [the] relationship in which a professional is identified as knowing well' (Lazega in Seabrooke 2014:4). This highlights the way in which knowledge claims and those who know well (the arbiters) are products of the relations underwriting Global AIDS, this being the process through which the 'cognitive authority' of certain actors is created (Broome and Seabrooke 2015:959). More specifically, these interests are linked with the global policy interests of international policy actors such as the UNAIDS, PEPFAR and the Gates Foundation that have emerged to deal with AIDS, and the way in which these organisations deploy biomedical knowledge and expertise as policy technology. Through these relations, arbiters become 'central nodes in the network, [who] can create "black boxes" that reinforce what knowledge is most appropriate and should not be questioned (Seabrooke 2014 13; Latour 1987). This is an important observation because it highlights critically how policy considerations in Global AIDS have become both limited and limiting. It also suggests that most participants in these conferences reproduce a form of solidarity with the AIDS community by being there, while also absorbing the knowledge provided by the arbiters.

5.3 How Then Does the Conferencing Work?

I will look now at some examples to highlight how conferencing works not only as a process of reproducing solidarity but also as a space within which the politics of knowledge is at work in reproducing the meta-framing of HIV and AIDS through a broadly biomedical lens. I argue that through mechanisms of participation and practices of knowledge presentation at conferences, state of the art knowledge is diffused.

The way in which the IAS conferences work can be observed in the following statement given by Deborah Birx, the Coordinator of the United States Government Activities to Combat HIV/AIDS. Here interview was given in Melbourne during the AIDS 2014a conference in Melbourne. She states that

> Over the last 48–72 hours it is exciting to see people are coalescing around the same concepts whether you are an advocate or whether you are a scientist or whether you are a clinician. The interest in making sure that people are undetectable to control the virus is the very essence of how they get to control the epidemic. To find how much alignment there is and goals and understanding where the gaps are. I think UNAIDS Gap report is extraordinary. It shows us where to go and we are all coalescing around young women, and paediatric treatment and need to get viral load access in resource-poor settings. So it is exciting (AIDS 2014a).

Birx's interview offers a summary of the way in which the conference space is used to reproduce solidarity and to create a common direction for different actors within the Global AIDS community. Given that the interview is given by someone who occupies a position of power within the Global AIDS system, it acts as a reassertion of the politics of knowledge as epistemic arbitrage discussed above. The language used to indicate common ground and common directions is important in giving directions to other actors to follow. Furthermore, it recognizes the knowledge claims in UNAIDS work as the relevant basis from which to develop future directions for the Global AIDS response. All of this, through the various priorities that are spelled out, recognizes implicitly the cognitive authority of the biomedical knowledge that underwrites the UNAIDS approach.

This process of setting out the kind of knowledge that is seen as relevant begins with the selection processes on who should be involved in the formal scientific program of the conference. This process itself is a public relations activity within the Global AIDS community itself because many constituents' needs will have to be addressed by inclusion in the formal programme. As with every conference, applicants are selected through procedures of application, evaluation and then selection by five scientific track committees: A – Basic and Translational Research, B – Clinical Research, C – Epidemiology and Prevention Research, D – Social and Political Research, Law, Policy and Human Rights, and E – Implementation Research, Economics, Systems and Synergies with other Health and Development Sectors (AIDS 2016a). This kind of differentiation is standard in conference organizing. The interesting issue here though is the way in which this filtering process is also about compartmentalizing and channelling AIDS knowledge according to the biomedical scaffolding that frames knowledge needs in this area. The first three tracks are entirely bio-medically orientated and between them establish the bulk of the conference proceedings. The other two tracks bring non-biomedical knowledge into the conference through the categories that tie them into the overall biomedical scaffolding. Track E offers a good example of this where inclusion is evaluated according to the utility of knowledge according to the policy implementation needs identified for biomedical developments. This explicitly presents the position that biomedical knowledge is the main driver of policy thinking. Other sources of knowledge are valorised only in relation to their utility within these already formed policies. Track D becomes the *containment category* both to show that Global AIDS is engaging with social sciences but also to limit both implicitly and structurally engagement to the priority issues established within the biomedical scaffolding. From a policy perspective, this then establishes a division between the first three tracks as the main sources of knowledge for global policy debate and the latter tracks, which have more marginal utility under this view.

The issue of whether the social sciences should engage with the discussions emerging from biomedical sciences together on the same panel does not come into debate. Given that each track evaluates the abstracts to form the panel that makes up that part of the overall programme, there is an inevitable compartmentalization.[4]

[4] Given the discrepancy between the available space and the issues that need to be covered, the process of creating panels is an arduous task that attempts to be inclusive so that important topics are not left out from the conference programme. This also highlights how appearing on the pro-

It is hard if not impossible to find panels in which scientists from different disciplinary backgrounds (social and medical) take part in debate and reflect on the translation of scientific innovation into policy thinking. And yet, in many panels biomedical scientists speculate about policy relevance on the basis of more limited innovations they present.

By looking at the online abstract submission tutorial for the AIDS 2016a, b conference, one can understand this situation further.[5] The tutorial purports to guide people in developing their submissions and to enhance the quality of submissions received. It distinguishes between two pathways through the process. The category one abstract format is appropriate for broadly biomedical science research based abstracts, and the category two format is for reporting lessons learned from programmes, policy implementations and projects. Research-based abstracts are required to have a conclusion which clearly states 'the significance of your findings/ outcomes of your findings/outcomes of your study for HIV prevention, treatment, care and or support and future implications of the results'. The second abstract category has an added category on 'lessons learned', where the submission needs to include the outcomes of the intervention that is being considered and 'analytical approaches, evaluation of lessons learned and best practices with succinct description of the methods used. In addition please summarize any specific results that specifically support your conclusions of lessons learned and best practices' (AIDS 2016b).

While this guidance may be helpful to prospective participants and abstract evaluators, it also provides a mechanism to encourage researchers to think about their work in relation to implementation science in regards to Global AIDS. Crucially, research output is framed in terms of its utility within the Global AIDS system. Given these conditions, the politics of AIDS surrounding these conferences is often reduced to attempts by social scientists to be included within the decision making process so as to influence change from within the Global AIDS system. Thus, success is often talked about as an attempt to influence how to name tracks, symposia and panels, or to facilitate the inclusion of more social scientists in what appear to be biomedical debates. Generally speaking, this has limited results. The social sciences may indeed appear in many discussions as a topic and there may even be a number of people who participate as social scientists in these debates. However, their inclusion is often little more than a public relations gesture to preserve the idea of the AIDS community within the Global AIDS system. It is also a selective process reflecting the bias observed by Kippax and Holt towards social scientists discussing individual behaviour. Let me provide two brief examples of this.

The first example comes from the AIDS 2012c conference. On Thursday 27 July 2012, the plenary panel discussion of the day in the central hall, included presentations from Paul Semigoma from Uganda on MSM and HIV looking at the health

---

gramme can become a political process independent of the abstract submission and selection procedures. Space for social sciences is even more limited within the more regional conferences that are organized between the biennial meetings.

[5] See http://www.aids2016.org/Programme/Abstracts/Submitting-your-abstract

implications of the Ugandan anti-homosexuality bill, Cheryl Overs from Australia who presented her work with sex workers and harm reduction, Debbie McMillan from Washington DC who talked about her experiences as a transgender women with HIV who is also a specialist working with Transgender Health Empowerment group, and Gottfried Hirnschall from WHO talking about the need to expand testing and treatment access. The panel was an example of the way in which the conference organizes a plenary session to begin each day which includes a mixture of biomedical scientists, policy makers and activists who present their work on a particular topic. The design of these sessions is not based on abstract submissions buts reflects the views of the conference organizing committee's members, the different voices they would like to include, and the issues they would like to highlight. This particular panel was no different. It included people who represented important issues that were of concern to the conference: the criminalization of sex between men and sex work, issues of relevance to transgender people, and treatment access. All the speakers provided important insights from their work and the problems they had observed. In one way though, it was perhaps a little different from some of the other panels in that Debbie McMillan's speech was one of the most moving speeches given at the audience. As she spoke about her early life experience as a transgender woman, it was clear that many in the audience were trying to hold back tears. This was the first plenary speech given by a transgender person at an IAS conference. In talking about herself, she provided an extraordinary mapping of socio-cultural, political and economic life in Washington DC, which had influenced her own life, her choices and her experiences:

> Welcome to the United States, we've missed you for the last 22 years. I want to specially thank IAS for giving me this opportunity to talk to you all, it's a privilege. Who am I, like most people the sum of who I am is much more than my individual traits. However, there are facts. They categorize me as high-risk in the HIV world. I am an African-American, I am a transgender woman, I used to be a drug user, I used to be a sex worker, I used to be incarcerated. For 20 years I lived a life that virtually guaranteed I would contact HIV. That should mean that I was then, or am now, irrelevant. That would greatly underestimate me and miss an opportunity to address HIV. I am here today because I represent people at the heart of the AIDS crisis, a small group with a big problem. If this is true then it should be equally true that the solution lies with people like me. When people like me are included in the design of policy and programing, these programs are much more successful. They are much less so when we are not consulted…I went to the street alone at 14. It seemed to be only place for someone like me. I became a commercial sex worker because I believed that was the only occupation for someone like me. I got high to dull the reality of the things I had to do to survive life.

After talking about the impact of drug use on HIV infection rates and the ways in which drug use and sex work are interlinked as a 'power and money relationship', Debbie went on to talk about the criminal justice system:

> No matter how risky life is outside, being in prison is worse. After one of many arrests for prostitution I was sent to a men's prison. I was housed in a wing with murderers and rapists. I am sure you can guess what happened. Nothing is gained by describing those details. I could have gotten HIV anywhere. But I am convinced I got it in prison… Instead of helping young … the American legal system punishes them in a way that significantly increases the chance of HIV infection. If you really look hard at drug addiction you will see that it is just

> a symptom, for me it was the stigma I experienced for most of my life as a transgender woman… My mother, an avid drug user and a sex worker, left me with my grandmother. For some, my mother represents everything that is wrong with America: someone who could have risen above her circumstances stayed in school but chose drugs and prostitution. For some, she represents the failure of the society to take care of the most vulnerable among us. To me, my mother was the only person who ever completely accepted me as I am. Unlike my mother my father disowned me when it became clear that my sexuality was not what he thought it should be. On the streets I look for acceptance, a family, a man who would give me what my father never did. At some point my mother was infected with HIV. While she was still alive and living with my grandmother she had one cup, one fork, one spoon, one plate; when she used the bathroom my grandmother followed behind her bleached everything she touched. During one of my incarcerations for solicitation my mother died of complications of AIDS. I had to view my mother's body alone in shackles and handcuffs. Two months later I was diagnosed with HIV. I was 20 years old and I was convinced I was going to die. So there I was, stigma on top of stigma.
>
> As a rule medical personnel don't excel in bedside manners when it comes to transgender people. It is hard enough to face HIV. You want a doctor who understands that your entire life changes when you get that diagnosis, not someone who does not bother to look at you in the eye to see the very basics of who you are (AIDS 2012c).

McMillan's presentation skillfully presented her life as being at the intersection of the HIV epidemic and the policy interventions that have attempted to deal with it in the USA. Her narrative offered both a critique and an evaluation of the common ground that has emerged on AIDS. Her evaluation challenged some of the assumptions about the ways in which the 'constituent elements' of a given life and AIDS interact 'in precisely predictable ways' to allow existing interventions to deal with the identified AIDS problem (Woolcock 2013: 234). McMillan's narrative presents life as having a, 'high causal density' in the form of multilayered interactive circumstances underpinning a

> '… high uncertainty which is a function of the numerous pathways and feedback loops connecting inputs, actions and outcomes, the entity's openness to exogenous influences, and capacity of constituent elements (most notably people) to exercise discretion (i.e. to act independently of or in accordance with rules, expectations, precedent, passions, professional norms or self-interest)' (Woolcock 2013:235).

This view offers a direct challenge to the biomedical gaze that tries to identify a general similarity among those impacted upon by AIDS so as to mount a technical policy response. It also challenges attempts to focus on individual behaviour as either an explanatory heuristic or the target of policy interventions independent of the life she describes.

The challenge highlights a set of socio-cultural, political, economic and psychological pathways that differentially locate individuals and their experiences of HIV with particular results. Furthermore, it also suggests that AIDS interventions and policies based on abstract categories (such as transgender or MSM) will have limited impact if they do not take into account the particular dynamics of the high causal density that makes life. This is also the challenge posed by the social and political sciences to the biomedical gaze. However, there was no clear attempt in this panel or in the conference more generally to understand the kind of analytical lens this narrative provides to think about AIDS from the position of life in all its dynamic interactions. And while the conference organizers may have considered McMillan's inclusion as an essential part of AIDS solidarity with transgender people, the conference's overarching biomedical stance viewed her presentation not as an analytic device, but as an 'occasion for tears' and a motivational speech to generate further support for the need to tackle AIDS with a particular key population or risk group in mind.

A second example comes from this same conference and took the form of a symposium panel held on Tuesday 24 July 2012. The panel was designed to launch a special issue of the journal the *Lancet* on HIV in men who have sex with men and HIV. This was an important intervention to focus attention on the state of affairs in relation to gay and other men who have sex with men globally. The panel took place in the same massive auditorium as the plenary sessions. It was scheduled for the afternoon and the auditorium was reasonably busy although not as full as it was for the plenary discussed above. The panel was chaired by the editor of the *Lancet*, Richard Horton, and Chris Beyrer. It was designed to include contributors to the *Lancet* special issue. There were seven presenters: Stefan D. Baral, Patrick Sullivan, Kenneth Mayer, Gregorio Millet, Chris Collins (all medicine and public health specialists from the USA), Gift Trapence (a community worker and activist from Malawi) and Dennis Altman (a social and political scientist from Australia). While it was clear that the panel was an attempt to be inclusive, its main focus was to look at the issue from a medical, epidemiological and public health perspective by talking about MSM in general, in a global context. Their concerns were implicitly organized around the notion of there being generic MSM individuals whose major characteristics could be framed by common behavioural considerations. Within this framing, Trapence's presentation focused on experiences of community engagement in Malawi. Only Altman offered a more nuanced account in thinking about homophobia that would allow engagement with men who have sex with men (gay or otherwise) in non-western socio-political settings. The overall MSM categorization that underwrote much of the discussion was tangential to the way in which Altman described the socio-political and cultural contexts of homophobia and its implications for global programming. This divergence of opinion is also observable in the structure of the *Lancet* special issue itself, which is divided into four sections: a comments section which includes several short pieces from community groups discussing the issues as they see them, and then a series of seven articles detailing bio-medical research on the issue. The only social science contribution is included in a separate section entitled 'Viewpoint' (Altman et al. 2012). While this situation may be explained away on the basis of the publication modalities of the Lancet as a medical journal, it still is perplexing given the centrality of the social science contribution to most of the other pieces in the special issue. Looking at the debate, it is clear that many of the articles map out the problems men who have sex with men face in different contexts – including disease dynamics, infection rates and access to treatment – with the goal of proposing somewhat generic policy directions. But, they display little social scientific understanding, using general terms such as lack of human rights and homophobia without paying close attention to what these mean, and how they manifest themselves in particular contexts influencing everyday lives.

The approach also highlights the limited interest other authors show in the social science article published in the same issue, which provides a more nuanced and grounded discussion of the issues.[6] Together with the panel discussion itself, it was clear that engagement with the social science position was both narrow and rhetorical. All the speakers clearly recognized the widely varying social, political and legal factors that enhance men who have sex with men's vulnerability to HIV within particular contexts. They recognized too that the term MSM is a something of a catch-all category, and that many different kinds of men are included within in. But, when thinking how best to deal with this situation, discussion switched back to how a generic health solution might work for the generic category of MSM globally. This pattern of thinking was uncannily similar to that observed in the case of the first example. It reveals an interest in socio-political issues but refuses to employ a social science analysis to engage with them.

This framing is also the mechanism that seeks to turn social and political research into the handmaiden of biomedicine via the trope of implementation science. Here, biomedical knowledge prescribes the best way of acting through the technologies of intervention that underwrite global policy thinking. Lock and Nguyen argue that the 'legitimation of biomedical technologies involves the dissemination of rhetoric about their value; at the most fundamental level, it is assumed that they contribute to scientific progress and further, that they fulfill human "needs"' (2010:23). Of course, what is implicit here is the way in which regardless of individual and social diversity human needs are assumed to be similar. What are established as needs are thereby attributed to all the identified members of a category, be this a sex worker, a transgender person or MSM. The people concerned thereby become the object of these technologies in policy thought. Social science thinking and a social science sensibility is rarely part of the development of this knowledge or the policies that follow from it. Arguably, by restricting the analytic concerns of the social sciences to implementation, a bias is created 'toward designing and improving one aspect of the policy process and implicitly suggests ignoring others' (O'Toole, Jr 2004: 313). As McMillan's speech on transgender experience and Altman's discussion of the cultural specificities of homophobia reveal, AIDS is as much a problem of race, class, religion and economic relations as it is a public health problem.

I will turn now to an interview given by Christopher Beyrer on 23 July 2012 during the AIDS 2012d Conference in Washington DC. The interview is important because it highlights some of the dynamics I have just discussed. Also, because Beyrer is a well-established medical scientist who became the President of IAS

[6] I am sure number of readers will be rather critical of this analysis, saying that it was important for this paper to be included in the *Lancet* special issue, and that it provided space to bring the social sciences into the discussion. I agree. However, this kind of tactical engagement speaks volumes about the politics of AIDS within the IAS conference, offering social science only the most limited space for engagement. Witnessing such an approach in practice provides little encouragement to other social scientists to engage with the issues in an open minded and critical manner, given that what one observes is in effect a practice of disciplining.

from 2014 to 2016, the interview provides some dramatic insights into what kind of knowledge counts within the Global AIDS system.

> Interviewer (I)-The conference's logo is about turning the tide together what do you think about that what does it mean to you?
>
> C. Beyrer (CB)- The tide is, of course, the tide of ever expanding AIDS epidemic. What we want to see in that turning is declines in infections. I think a very realistic goal is dramatic reductions close to eradication of paediatric HIV infections. I think many people believe that that is the most achievable of these goals. To me as an epidemiologist who has worked in many different countries, but spending quite a bit of time in Russia and Central Asia, I have to say that that component of the global epidemic is expanding, is not going in the direction of turning the tide and I think reasons for that are mostly because of the challenges with Russia and with most of the states of Former Soviet Union to adopt evidence-based programmes and policies for people who inject drugs and people who are at sexual risk. I don't see any evidence that we are beginning to turn that tide. So I would say when we think turning the tide together to me it means the whole world is going to have to do this.
>
> We have a similar problem with the epidemic among gay and bisexual men or men who have sex with men. The rates are rising in many countries including developed countries with good health systems with good access to health care. So that's another component of the epidemic that is expending in 2012 and we now really have to address.
>
> I-What is your message?
>
> CB-I really think that what we can begin to use this extraordinary moment of optimism we now have to work together as a global community, researchers, policy makers, the community of people affected to start really to make these gains, the recent scientific gains real for people on the ground. This conference is going to be about how we implement the exciting new science and really put it to use and the very critical question will we do that? Do we have still the political will to do this? Are we going to be able to fight the donor fatigue? Are we going to be able to do this in the context of very tough times for donor countries particularly in Western Europe? I hope answer to all those questions is yes. But I think a big part of what this conference is about asking those questions.
>
> I-According to you what is the biggest obstacles to turn the tide right now?
>
> CB-I think the single biggest obstacle is really going to be the challenges of providing necessary evidence-based services and human rights services for people who in so many societies remain excluded. These are what sometimes called more at risk populations and sometimes called key populations. But what we are talking about is sexual minorities, men who have sex with men, sex workers, people who use drugs and particularly people who inject drugs. Those populations continue to be under served, under resourced and we are not going to turn the tide in HIV unless they are truly included and that is going to be an enormous challenge. That has been since the beginning of AIDS and still is (AIDS 2012d).

As a passionate scientist and activist, Beyrer's interview shows how his thinking is located within the broader set of understandings that underpin Global AIDS knowledge as a conceptual system. He systematically highlights the way in which a number of issues are major concerns for Global AIDS. At the same time, he points to the future when he talks of biomedical 'scientific gains', 'making these gains real for people on the ground' and using 'evidence based programmes and policies'. The idea of making gains real here is about bringing scientific technologies to people globally. The possibility of doing this successfully rests on treating people with AIDS categorically as policy targets whose needs are identified from a similar knowledge base. The idea of being on the ground points to the difference between the scientific knowledge that matters and the 'ground' as a generic context of implementation, be it the states of the post-Soviet Union or the developed countries of

Africa and Asia. The challenging circumstances that influence the concerns identified by Beyrer as relevant to gay, bisexual and other men who have sex with men are brought together as a subject area that shows a similarity of needs. The success of this framing is achieved linguistically by framing all of these issues as 'a component of the epidemic' that 'we now really have to address' from the Global AIDS perspective.

In recognizing the global structural issues of funding and leadership, Beyrer's real concern seems to be about maintaining the delivery of what we think will work. In discussing obstacles, he identifies socio-political and economic problems as obstacles for people who inject drugs and with marginalized sexualities to have access to what we know works. What is clear here is the way in which socio-political and economic conditions are not considered at all in relation to how HIV emerges as a particular kind of health problem in different settings at the intersections of socio-political, economic and psychological conditions. Beyrer's account seems to suggest that these conditions are problems *we* need to overcome to engage with the disease as *we* identify it. Furthermore, as he says 'the tide in HIV' will not be turned 'unless they are truly included'; the implicit idea here being that 'being included' seems to be about being included in the Global AIDS system and in the way it chooses to frame HIV and AIDS as problems.

This is interesting as it points to a refusal to understand the constitutive link between what is considered an 'AIDS problem' and the socio-political and economic conditions he identifies. I would argue that this situation derives from not looking at these problems and their causes from the analytical stance that could be provided by the social and political sciences. Without such an analysis, arguing for evidence-based programmes and policies to overcome these obstacles rather misses the point, ignoring entirely the social conditions that inform particular experiences of being, acting, and experiencing HIV. It is this thinking that reduces the dynamic causal complexity discussed above into being a member of an abstract AIDS policy target category. The interview, as a part of the conference context, sets out clearly how knowledge actors, or arbiters, in the Global AIDS system frame both debate and set out future horizons for other participants.

One final example in this context comes from an interview given by the executive director of *AVAC – Global Advocacy for HIV Prevention,* Mitchell Warren, on 24 July 2014 during the AIDS 2014a, b, c in Melbourne. He was asked to discuss major issues that occupy the policy actors and activists around the conference. His response was as follows.

> Within these conferences every two years there is really every possible issue under the sun, every conference is a turning point, every conference takes us into a new direction. But I think we are at a point that two years ago in Washington everyone was talking about, ending the epidemic that was coming out of the HPTN 052 study, this idea that treatment was not only treatment but can also have preventative benefits. So we are here two years later and the buzz is UNAIDS before the conference we should end the epidemic by 2030. And that is absolutely the …goal but how do we get there you know you don't just determine the goal and go on an auto-pilot. You need to be incredibly intentional. There is a huge amount of work about delivering things we have and the treatment is the backbone of that. And condom use, behaviour change communication things we have done for 30 years with

> prevention and the last 20 years with treatment, we need to do all of that and more, increasing the scale and the pace. But there is an essential need to do other things too. So this is an interesting meeting in that seeing the scale of the main stream interventions in treatment and prevention and amazing, I think, new success story of voluntary medical male circumcision a biomedical intervention with a huge behavioural, social and cultural control component demonstrating to work 7 years ago in clinical trials and now finally we are seeing the impact. Similarly oral pre-exposure prophylaxis is now proven 4 years ago by iPrEX results come out on men who have sex with men, FDA approved it 2 years ago, and in the last two months we have CDC and WHO guidelines really telling us as a matter of fact that PrEP is the real deal. PrEP has a role in combination prevention. But how do you roll it out, who wants it, who will use it and we are beginning to see in this meeting first time real data to tell us that, although we know PrEP is not for everyone PrEP is for some people, some of the time can have an important impact. So that is the kind of this middle level if we bring all the mainstream stuff … how do you demonstrate the added benefit of circumcision and PrEP. And then in this meeting too there is the wide long term development agenda which is really better therapies, vaccine and cure so you have all of them playing you really have to figure out if we are going to get to 2030 deliver what we've got, demonstrate this added benefit of newer interventions and never lose sight of the long term end game strategy of vaccine and cure that's going to be critical (AIDS 2014b).

Here, Warren enthusiastically talks about the central issues for Global AIDS by framing these as broadly biomedical developments and related solutions. His orientation locates the possibility of ending the epidemic in the potential created by biomedical interventions and their scaling up. His language here is of *us and we*, underwriting a certain solidarity within this community but at the same time clearly locating the possibility of further biomedical developments and related policy thinking in resource-rich settings. Later in his interview, Warren acknowledges structural issues such as stigma and criminalization. I will discuss this more fully in the final chapter, but it is sufficient here to say that his approach to these issues seems to consider them as structural problems preventing the imaginary 'us' from delivering what we know works.

5.4 Conclusion

Throughout this chapter I have argued that the Global AIDS system frames the nature of the knowledge that it considers to be relevant for its policy practices. This framing is guided by two significant aspects of the Global AIDS system: the way in which AIDS emerged as a biomedical concern, and the global policy need to address HIV in and across multiple contexts. Both of these elements are legitimated by the solidarity claims of the AIDS movement that underpin the Global AIDS system and its right to deal with HIV and AIDS globally.

The chapter has looked in detail at how the politics of knowledge is reproduced within the Global AIDS system by reproducing the competency of certain actors – most usually biomedical scientists and those policy actors who can participate in international debates – to produce and diffuse knowledge. I have argued that the issue here is not only about biomedicine versus the social sciences and how this divide medicalizes AIDS discussion, but also about the way in which biomedical assumptions about human beings and their health frame the entirety of knowledge needs and policy directions on HIV and AIDS. It is also about how this meta-framing gives credibility to the policy implementation strategies and the related success claims of the global system.

In this process, HIV-related knowledge as a part of the mechanisms of reproduction of the Global AIDS system maintains a system of thinking and knowledge production process that 'gives weight to an "internalizing" discourse even when its acknowledgement of factors that are external to the body may well be at least in part contributory to the condition' (Lock and Nguyen 2010: 61). This leads to solutions that target diverse bodies with HIV as if they were one. The role of these bodies, in this process, is simply to adhere to what has been given to them through HIV-related policy intervention, and the lives that these bodies represent are reduced to having access to settings in which they can encounter, take up and use prescribed Global AIDS interventions. This ignores the everyday social processes that allow people to 'make sensible choices in congealing problem-solving round a complex, context-specific, and dynamic' problems such as HIV and AIDS (O'Toole Jr 2004:314). In turn, it leads to framing the concerns of Global AIDS in terms of bodies with HIV, where HIV becomes the commonality that drives policy thinking rather than HIV as encountered by a diversity of people in a variety of ways and in varying circumstances. This homogenizing approach is legitimated by the way in which a biomedical approach focuses on the 'material body, the assumption of a universal body, and the associated idea that illness is deviation about a standardized "norm", all contribute to the assertion of a moral position' (Lock and Nguyen 2010: 58).

This delimitation has critical implications for Global AIDS as a policy system. It not only establishes how biomedical thinking approaches HIV, but it also portrays biomedicine as the master epistemological frame within which to include social facts relevant to dealing with the epidemic. It creates both a spurious uniformity about HIV and about the social body that needs to respond to the disease. It is through this kind of thinking that social science concerns are incorporated, by reducing them to categorical concerns, for instance, on gender, on MSM or on safe sex, as 'solutions' to be implemented by the universal social body that responds to AIDS. Implementation science is the way in which this uniform social response is to be achieved. As O'Toole Jr argues, by focusing the social sciences on implementation science, the Global AIDS system creates 'a bias towards one form of system design or redesign rather than another' (2004:313). In this way, Global AIDS reduces the social sciences to meeting its engineering needs within different settings. This reduction is essentially about externalizing the complex social dynamics of personal and everyday life by filtering these first to the social facts that matter in relation to HIV, and then to those *we* need to alter in order to deal with HIV in general.

In some ways, this process is informed by a logic of 'looking for and finding', in which the looking for points to what might be described as an 'intentional' orientation (Descombes 2014:83). The categorical approach adopted by the Global AIDS system, both in terms of risk groups and the relevant social facts about them, constitutes the process of looking for. Both researchers and policy actors also act 'under description' (Anscombe 2000). Their thinking is limited with the way in which Global AIDS system has already mapped out the problems, the solutions and the means of getting to them. As I have argued throughout this chapter, this is only possible because Global AIDS itself creates the spaces and the processes within them whereby this cognitive mapping appears 'to individuals themselves, in discussion between them, in a dialogical way' (Descombes 2014: 92). IAS conferences and the examples I have cited in this chapter reveal aspects of this dialogical process in reproducing the meanings (solidarity, global disease and others) assigned to AIDS, in diffusing these meanings, and in guiding action (knowledge production and policy thinking) for all the participants under the guise of solidarity. While this leads to ever increasing internalization of social concerns within the dominant Global AIDS viewpoint, it also further abstracts social and political concerns from the everyday contexts in which people live, and directs attention away from experience-based knowledge about what really matters – both socially and politically – within a given context. Without doubt, this has important policy implications for the sustainability of many HIV-related interventions in people's everyday lives.

Chapter 6
Evidence-Based Policy: *Randomised Controlled Trials'* Knowledge Claims to AIDS Policy

In this chapter, I intend to explore why knowledge claims based on Randomised Controlled Trial (RCT) evidence has been so favoured by high level Global AIDS actors to justify decision-making and related policy development. The aim here is to deepen the analysis provided by the last chapter by looking at one specific policy instance and examining how the knowledge that was seen as relevant to this case was produced. I will also look at how Global AIDS itself creates the justification for the further use of RCTs to justify the policy relevance of its knowledge claims in general.

The need to provide a close reading of the links between knowledge production and policy development is justified by the number of times biomedical knowledge claims seem to have guided policy directions in the examples considered in the last chapter. Chris Beyrer, for example, explicitly talked about making '[these] gains, the recent scientific gains real for people on the round'. Mitchell Warren, in turn, talked about 'delivering [the] things we have' described some of these gains as success stories demonstrated through trials. These included the HPTN 052 trial which led to the development of treatment as prevention policy, the 'amazing success of voluntary medical male circumcision (VMMC) [as] demonstrated to work in clinical trials', and more recently the iPrEX trial demonstrating the efficacy of oral pre-exposure prophylaxis (PrEP) against HIV. Each of these statements points to how biomedical trial results offer the basis for policy making within a Global AIDS approach. Once trials suggest that a particular intervention works, they resolve the question of what to do for policy purposes. The remaining policy problem here is not about the knowledge and its limits, but about having enough resources to bring the right biotechnical tools to those who need them.

One of the specific questions I want to consider in this chapter is to what extent one can legitimately develop global policy on HIV based on the findings from a specific RCT conducted in a particular context? Asking this question allows me to navigate a number of issues central to this debate: (a) understanding the conditions and the kind of knowledge RCTs produce; (b) understanding the conditions of generalizability of this knowledge; and (c) unpacking the relationship between

H. Seckinelgin, *The Politics of Global AIDS*, Social Aspects of HIV 3,
DOI 10.1007/978-3-319-46013-0_6

knowledge claims provided by a given RCT and the way these are later used by policy actors. But, before I turn to substantive discussion of these issues, however, I want to briefly provide an overview of the emergence of RCT debate in general and its relevance to one of the main concerns of this book: namely, the impact of the Global AIDS system in framing knowledge production practices for AIDS policy.

S. Lochlann Jain has described the medical RCT in its simplest form as a trial

> ...in which one group of patients would receive the new treatment and the other group would be given the standard treatment. No one would know which group they were in until the end of the trial, at which time the survivors would be counted, the side effects measured, a decision made about whether to take the drug to the next stage. (2010: 89; also see Lambert 2009)

In more technical terms, Nancy Cartwright considers the kind of causal claim inherent in the knowledge produced in this process, when she writes,

> Knowledge like this involves a [third kind of] causal claim, a power or capacity claim: the treatment reliably promotes the outcome, or reliably contributes across a given range of circumstances. "Reliably promotes" means roughly that across a wide range of circumstances there will be more cases, or a higher level, of the outcome with the treatment than there would be without it. What the actual numbers are depends on what other factors are present. (2011: 1401)

Margaret Lock and Vinh-Kim Nguyen in their analysis of the emergence of experimental methodology and RCTs, trace this process back to the possibilities opened up by 'the idea of biological commensurability' which 'allows people to be sorted into standardized groups and populations because the[ir] biology is assumed to be the same' (2010: 176). Their definition of biological commensurability suggests that this process is less about making all bodies the same, than the creation of conventions to make them comparable and thus measurable against each other. They state that biological commensurability

> ...establishes a set of agreed-upon rules about how the body is assumed to work, and furnishes a series of hypothetical equivalences, for example that a liver, a stem cell, or a chromosome is biologically equivalent in all human bodies. Human biology becomes, then, a yardstick that can be used to measure difference in terms of variation about a norm, and in this way bodies are made commensurable. (2010:177)

Such an understanding highlights a number of important issues relevant to the ongoing discussion. Of particular interest is (i) how the development of experimentation (as a research method) and its development into RCT procedures connects with particular needs and contexts; (ii) how such processes reflect attempts to control the health of populations under particular political regimes; and (iii) how the political nature of these approaches disappears as debate becomes more focused on developments to increase the technical accuracy of these experimental processes rather than the uses to which they are out (Lock and Nguyen 2010:176–188). Of significance too is how the nature of this approach and the policies resulting from it, become focused on individual bodies and their functions. Through such an approach, individual bodies with HIV or at risk of acquiring HIV become key populations in relation to the Global AIDS approach and its recommended interventions.

Through their use over time, RCTs have come to dominate evidence-based medicine (EBM) and evidence-based policy (EBP), providing a Gold Standard approach to knowledge creation relevant to particular populations. The method has also come to influence work in other fields. For example, the use of RCTs in economics is discussed in an influential article by Joshua D. Angrist and Jorn-Steffen Pischke (2010). The authors strongly endorse the method, arguing that 'such studies offer a powerful method for deriving results that are defensible both in the seminar room and in a legislative hearing' (2010: 4). In their conclusions, they argue that 'empirical work in this spirit has produced a credibility revolution in the fields of labour, public finance and development economics over the past 20 years' (2010:26).

In development economics, the work of Abhijit Banerjee and Esther Duflo is also considered highly influential. They argue that the

> ...field experiment emerged as an attractive new tool in [efforts] to elaborate our understanding of economic issues relevant to poor countries and poor people. By enabling the researcher to precisely control the variation in data, field experiments allow the estimation of parameters and testing of hypotheses that would be very difficult to implement with observational data. (Banerjee and Duflo 2010:62)

The movement of the RCT method from medicine to economics is not accidental. Michael P. Keane argues that 'economic empiricists regard the randomized control trails conducted in medicine as the "Gold Standard"' (2010: 55). This view can readily be observed in discussions where RCT success as a general experimental method is highlighted before their use in economics is discussed (see, for example, List 2010: 3 and Ludwig, Kling and Mullainathan 2011: 33).

RCT method has become attractive to HIV-related policy thinking for number of reasons. First, it offers a style of research which is closely aligned with the biomedical thinking that has framed the Global AIDS system. It is assumed to provide a properly 'scientific' justification for the policies developed (Lock and Nguyen 2010: 187–188). More pragmatically in the Global AIDS field, policy makers seem to accept what many RCT advocates claim as an advantage of the method: namely, that it shows *what works* as an intervention. It is self-evident for most policy makers to focus their funding and efforts on what works, rather than on interventions that are untested and/or have not been proven to work.

The claim to being scientific is based on the technical procedures used in constructing and then running a RCT: in particular its use of experimental and control groups, and the analysis of findings using mathematical and statistical methods. This situation satisfies two needs of the Global AIDS system simultaneously – endorsing the value of the medical model which considers people with HIV as comparable biological objects, while providing policy formulations to address donor concerns for reach, efficiency and global policy impact.[1]

---

[1] HIV and AIDS investment represents one of the biggest single issues here, with 16.11 billion US dollars being spent in 2011 (UNAIDS 2012) within international development. The nature of HIV interventions, in particular treatment roll-out, requires a gradual increase in this funding over time. Therefore, many donors are looking for cost-effectiveness in interventions to reach the widest beneficiary groups.

Of course, RCT methodology has also been the subject of much debate (see, for example, Cohen and Easterly 2009; Rodrik 2009; Ravallion 2009; Barrett and Carter 2010; Deacon 2010; Harrison 2011; Shaffer 2011; Cartwright and Hardie 2012; Teele 2014). Considering the critical discussion that has taken place within the field of international development economics where RCT method has come to dominate, it is in some ways surprising that in another international development related field, HIV and AIDS, the implications of these debates are rarely considered when RCT-based policy decisions are promoted or taken up (Banarjee and Duflo 2010). This highlights a major issue: while there has been robust defence of the method in terms of its general construction, concerns about external validity,[2] particularly for the development of general policy formulation, remain. Perhaps this is because the main justification for generalizability of the research outcomes derives from biological commensurability assumptions linking research to policy. This has led to a *(bio)social commensurability* that allows comparisons and evaluations of different social systems in relation to HIV. The relevance of the experimental knowledge which allows these steps to underwrite policy thinking is grounded by an emergency logic. As Adriana Petryna has observed, 'To what extent does the language of crisis become instrumental, granting legitimacy to experimentation when it otherwise might have none?' (2009: 35).

This question of external validity relates not only to the way in which trials are conducted but also to how their results are interpreted for policy concerns within the crisis framework provided by Global AIDS. Petryna goes on to argue that 'in zones of crisis, protection and safety considerations are at times weighed against immediate health benefits or the scientific knowledge to be gained' (2009: 36). Given that the Global AIDS system has framed HIV as a emergency, its policy approach is one of expediency to save lives. This position is observable when eminent AIDS actors suggest that the results of various RCT trials should lead to a generalized policy approach. The underlying logic here is that with good enough evidence from well-designed RCTs (itself an assumption) and biological commensurability underpinning HIV infection (another assumption), there can be no valid reason to hesitate in times of 'emergency' (yet another assumption) in developing generalizable policy guidelines and interventions. But there may be too many assumptions here to adequately bridge the gap between RCT results and the generalized policy advice that is based on them. Because of this, in Global AIDS discourse, RCT-based claims of 'what works' need to be carefully evaluated both for the veracity of the claims being made, and for their relevance to policy making.

In the rest of the chapter I want to analyze the relationship between one particularly influential RCT-based study in the HIV field, the claims it made, and the way in which a policy prescription was later developed. The aim here is to understand the way in which an RCT establishes a relationship between a particular intervention and a desired outcome within a given context, and how this research output is then linked to policy as evidence for implementation. The critical issue at stake is

[2] External validity concerns the extent to which the results of a study or experiment can be generalized to a wider population or a wider set of circumstances.

how the knowledge produced by an RCT is used, not only as evidence to justify a particular policy stance, but also as substantive policy content.

The trial I will focus on is the Routine versus Clinically Driven Laboratory Monitoring of HIV Antiretroviral therapy in Africa (DART) study and its reported output (Dart 2010). I have decided to use this particular case rather than looking at the more recent PrEP (Auerbach and Hoppe 2015; Buchbinder and Liu 2015; Cáceres et al. 2015; Kebaabetswe et al. 2014), or the Voluntary Male Circumcision (Boyle and Hill 2011; Wamai et al. 2012; de Camargo et al. 2013; Wamai et al. 2015; Parkhurst et al. 2015)[3] trials, partly because the latter are already well discussed (Boyle and Hill 2011; Wamai et al. 2012; de Camargo et al. 2013) and partly to focus on a case where biological commensurability rapidly equates to biosocial commensurability. The case in question highlights how the meta-epistemological governance of AIDS knowledge through preferred method choices is made by Global AIDS actors. The following section unpacks the kind of mechanisms represented in the particular knowledge claims made at the end of the trial. I then consider the way in which this knowledge and the mechanisms identified within it were transferred to policy thought as substantive areas of intervention to deal with HIV treatment in resource poor-settings.

6.1 An RCT to Consider Efficiency of Treatment Delivery

On 9 December 2009, the BBC News reported the results of a medical trial in Africa under the headline 'Scrap tests "to boost HIV care"' (2009). The news item stated that 'researchers concluded that thousands more people in Africa could be treated with anti-retroviral therapy (ART), the main treatment for HIV/AIDS, if routine lab monitoring was dropped'. The in-depth scientific report of this trial, entitled Routine versus Clinically Driven Laboratory Monitoring of HIV Antiretroviral therapy in Africa (DART): A randomized non-inferiority trial, was published in the *Lancet* on 9 January, 2010 (DART Trial Team 2010). In their introduction, the team leading the trial talk about their motivation for conducting the research. They point out that expanded ART roll-out in resource-poor settings where health and medical infrastructure are limited, such as in Africa, has produced new challenges. They identify one of these as the delivery of ART without being able to assess the potentially toxic effects of the delivered medications. They state that 'whether treatment programs should provide laboratory monitoring or focus resources on continuing to expand access to first-line and second-line ART is a crucial debate in the present economic crisis' (DART Trial Team 2010:123). But what is the 'economic crisis' being talked about here? Clearly, it is not the global economic crisis, as the trial itself pre-dated the 2008 economic crash. It is more likely what was then an emerging funding crisis

[3] I am providing the first four references here not to take part in the ongoing controversy these articles are presenting on VMMC. I think they are useful as they represent the depth and breath of the debate and literature on this topic.

in the HIV field. Although aid in this field had been substantial, at the time of the study the international trend in funding has been levelling. In real terms this represented a decline, as increased ART coverage increased the funding need together with the needs for additional interventions on care and prevention at the same time. This combination of factors appears to drive the reasons for the trial: to see whether an intervention that is at variance with the conventional ART delivery strategy in resource-rich countries might be efficacious in resource-poor settings in Africa. The trial team points out that, 'in resource-rich countries patients receiving ART have routine (typically every 3 months) tests to monitor efficacy and toxic effects. This testing is not mandated in public health ART rollout because it needs high-technology laboratory services and substantial resources' (DART Trial Team 2010:123).

The trial team's interest is in seeing whether this difference in delivery has an adverse effect on patients who are introduced to ART. They point out that 'if routine laboratory tests do not add significant benefit, ART programmes would be open to decentralization with long-term follow up in local clinics, rather than distant hospitals, providing that consistent and god quality care could be provided' (DART Trial Team 2010:123). They do not, however, entirely rule out the need for laboratory services as they argue that these 'could be targeted to assessment for ART eligibility and to diagnosis and management of opportunistic infections or clinical toxicity, rather than being done routinely' (2010:123). The DART trial is described as having been 'designed to investigate whether the delivery of ART with or without routine monitoring of CD-4 cell counts for efficacy, and haemotology and biochemistry for safety, [leads] to similar outcomes in HIV infected patients receiving ART who had already fulfilled clinical and CD-4 count criteria to start ART' (DART Trial Team 2010: 123).

The trial itself took place in two countries: in Uganda – at the Medical Research Council Unit in Entebbe, in the Joint Clinical Research Centre in Mulago, Kampala, and in Academic Alliances Clinic in Kampala; and in Zimbabwe at the University of Zimbabwe Research Centre in Harare. The team explain their procedure as being about 'randomly assigned to receive clinically driven monitoring (CDM) or laboratory plus clinical monitoring (LCM) for toxic effects (haematology and biochemistry) and efficacy (CD4-cell counts)' (DART Trial Team 2010:124). According to the procedure, 'all patients saw a doctor and had a routine blood count with white cell differential, lymphocyte tests at screening 4 and 12, and then every 12 weeks' (DART Trial Team 2010: 124). The LCM group doctors were given results of regular 3-monthly blood tests to check for ART drug-side effects and CD4-cell counts. The CDM group doctors received the same ART and regular blood test results but the results of safety tests were only provided if they were seriously abnormal (i.e. if the observed toxic effects were not within the safety criteria established) and CD4-cell counts were never seen. The important issue here is that both groups had direct access to required tests when and if the need arose in addition to required medical interventions as a result of these tests. Furthermore 'all participants received ART and were reviewed by a nurse every 4 weeks' (DART Trial Team 2010: 125). While providing all the required support the study aim was to see whether CDM was not inferior to a LCM-based intervention, and whether CDM instead of LCM could be used without the regular testing requirements associated with being on ART by relying on clinical observations. The trial involved a 'planned sample size of 3300 adults followed up for 4–6 years [to provide] 80 % power to establish that CDM was not inferior to LCM' (DART Trial Team 2010:125). The researchers explain that 'non-inferiority was defined as the upper 95 % confidence limit for the hazard ratio for new stage WHO stage 4 events or death being no greater than 1·18, which is equivalent to a yearly rate of progression of no more than 11·8 per 100 person-years in CDM compared with a predicated rate of 10·0 per 100 person years in LCM' (DART Trial Team 2010:125).

Some of the indicators used to assess how well the trial performed are important to the discussion here. The team's report points out that '234 (7 %) participants were lost to follow up'. It is not clear what the reason was for this; this might have been death-related but this is not known. Another observation relates to the nurse and doctor visits: 'completeness of nurse visits every 4 weeks and doctor visits every 12 weeks was high and similar in both groups (nurse visits 97.7 % in CDM *vs* 97.8 % in LCM group; doctor visits 98.7 % *vs* 98.8 %' (Dart Trial Team 2010:126). These high levels of visit frequency indicate the stringent procedures followed and the resources available to maintain these levels of engagement with participants over the trial period. Again it is stated that clinicians or nurses looking after participants in CDM element of the study could ask for laboratory tests if they deemed these necessary at any time. In addition, 'haematology or biochemistry panels could also be requested, if clinically indicated at intervening nurse visits every 4 weeks or extra patient-initiated visits in both groups (DART Trial Team 2010:126). These observations indicate the level of care-related control operationalized in the trail. They also reveal the availability of comprehensive medical and care resources to participants during the trials.

The team also reports on the CDM and LCM groups' ART status. They state that 'at Dec 31, 2008 or last clinic visit, 1346 (81 %) people receiving CDM versus 1295 (78 %) receiving LCM were still on first-line ART, including 288 (17 %) CDM and 281(17 %) LCM participants who had substituted one or more first-line drugs' (2010: 126). In the CDM group, 'overall 314 (19 %) people' received second-line ART in comparison to '361 (22 %) in the LCM group' (DART Trial Team 2010:127). In terms of the frequency of switching to second-line ART, they report that frequency was higher in the LCM group than the CDM group in the second and third years once participants started on ART (2010:127). Overall, they report that '459 (28 %) CDM participants versus 356 (21 %) LCM participants had a new WHO stage 4 event or died' (DART Trial Team 2010: 217). They also observe that 'new WHO stage 4 event-free survival at 5 years was 72 % (CI70-74) in the CDM group versus 78 % (76–80) in the LCM group and the number needed to monitor for 1 year to avoid one event was 59.62 % (408/654) of all new WHO stage 4 events and 65 % (248/382) of deaths occurred in the first 2 years' (DART Trial Team 2010:127). In explaining the differences between the CDM and LCM groups, the team points out that 'later switching leading to lower CD4-cell group in the CDM group was driving the difference among groups' (DART Trial Team 2010:127). In addition, with respect to the overall trends they state that

> Median CD4 counts for 2337 participants last seen alive on first-line ART was 339 cells per μL in the CDM group and 372 cells per μL in the LCM group, with 81 of 1178 (7 %) versus 22 of 1159 (2 %) respectively having CD4 counts less than 100 cells per μl. More CDM than LCM participants also had low CD4-cell counts at death on first-line treatment. (DART Trial Team 2010: 127)

These observations provide an interesting set of questions for the trial: was the difference in CD4 cell counts observed between the two groups while on first-line ART linked to the characteristics of participants allocated into two groups? Does the difference relate to the procedures used for testing for toxic effects in the two groups? And how best do we understand the large difference observed in the lower than 100 cells per μl CD4 counts in both groups? The report does not provide answers to these questions. In their discussion, the team come to a conclusion about the overall results of the trial in relation to the concern about the inferiority of CDM over LCM. They argue first that 'the results clearly show that first-line ART can be delivered safely without routine ... monitoring for toxic effects, but that routine CD4-cell count monitoring has a *small* but *significant benefit* in terms of disease progression and mortality, *probably* owing to slightly earlier switching to second-line ART' (DART Trial Team 2010: 128 *emphasis added*). The small but significant difference here indicates better survival opportunity for patients. The statement about probable reasons for the differences in disease progression and mortality shows that the team was not able to show clearly whether the switch to second-line medication, which allowed better treatment for some patients, was due only to CD4-cell count or the combined effect of such tests and the broader monitoring that involved testing for toxic effects (or, given that in the LCM more frequent tests were conducted, this too may have been a reason for the early-switch).

The trial sought to examine whether there would be an increase in disease progression and mortality with CDM compared to LCM. However, the investigators considered a limited increase acceptable on the basis of their definition of non-inferiority. This view of non-inferiority was justified in the study with regard to the costs involved in LCM-related tests and the lack of other resources: 'given the likely costs of routine laboratory monitoring, small differences would be unlikely to be cost effective and given the potential of CDM to allow wider ART rollout in Africa' (2010: 128). The actual reason stated here is the recognition that there is an opportunity cost for laboratory monitoring in dealing with patient treatment issues and ART roll-out more broadly.[4]

[4] Arguably, in an ideal resource-rich context, this dilemma should not occur. One would also argue that an implicit choice is being made on the assumption that it is impossible to improve resource infra-structure in Africa and therefore saving more lives is targeted by trying to increase the coverage of treatment independent of the other available medical resources. However, this does not deal with the increased need for medical resources due to bringing more people into ART treatment if the predicted decline in costs is achieved from not spending the resources on laboratories.

6.2 Why Does This Matter?

On 9 December 2009, the UK Medical Research Council's web page carried a statement from the co-principal investigator of this study, Professor Diana Gibb which read

> ...the survival of people who took part in the trial was remarkable: without treatment only about 10 % of HIV-infected African people like those in DART would be expected to survive for five years. In DART 87 % of those receiving treatment without routine blood test monitoring were still alive well after five years, only 3 percentage points less than in the group that had routine blood test monitoring. For health policy-makers in Africa, DART provides evidence that more people be treated for the same amount of money by not using routine laboratory tests. (MRC 2009)

It is worth pondering this statement carefully since it represents a move from research to policy prescription. It is particularly interesting claim to make, since both sides of the debate are linked by the one person who makes the statement: namely, the co-principal investigator. Furthermore in the move from the findings of a particular study conducted under specialized conditions in just two countries to policy prescription for 'health policy-makers in Africa', the findings are explicitly generalized.

The situation identified here highlights a particular relationship between research and policy making. Nancy Cartwright provides an analytic framework for understanding the mechanisms involved in the shift from particular research to general policy prescription. She points out that in policy statements similar to the one above, the move follows the sequence of identifying that something works in a particular context to making a statement that it works in general, which then allows the final step, namely, that it *will work for us* (Cartwright 2010). Here, it 'works in general' and it 'works for us' are implicit in the part of the statement that says '[F]or health policy-makers in Africa, DART provides evidence that more people be treated for the same amount of money by not using routine laboratory tests' (MRC 2009). This suggests that the findings are relevant for all of Africa, and that health policy makers across the continent should act on the basis of them if they wish to save money. The analytical modality captured by the formulation of it works here, it works in general, and it works for us, helps understanding of the distinct steps taken by researchers and policy makers when they link particular research findings to their own contexts and interest areas. Through such linkage, policy makers buy into the causal narrative constructed by the trial, which is implicit in the claim that *it works here*.

In a similar vein, the conditions under which any 'it works' statement holds true need to be carefully considered. For instance, we are told in the DART study that 'the results clearly show that first-line ART can be delivered safely without routine biochemistry and haemotology monitoring for toxic effects, but that routine CD4-cell count monitoring has a small but significant benefit in terms of disease progression and mortality, probably owing to slightly earlier switching to second-line ART' (DART Trial Team 2010: 128). If we take this as being correct, and if the difference created by CDM over LCM is not significant, then why does it matter whether it is inferior or not? In other words in terms of the assessment of inferiority, the result is not strong enough to justify under the experimental conditions a switch from LCM to CDM. Instead, it appears that the switch is justified as a result of the policy context within which the experiment was conducted: potentially declining aid budgets within the context of the growing need for more funding to support expanded ART roll-out. Here, the claim that something 'worked' in the trial presents an interpretation according to assumptions linked to the needs of international policy makers engaged in HIV policy making.

Looking at the argument more closely, it is interesting to note that the research findings highlight a particular trade-off between the routine testing for toxic effects which is expensive and the significantly higher costs attached to early switching of people in the CDM group to second-line drugs. Here, the issue is the fact that second-line drugs are much more expensive, and although LCM and its laboratory requirements are also expensive, since they allow selective switching to second-line drugs if and when tests require this, the LCM procedure seems to have the more efficient cost implications. However, the authors argue that

> …if budget constraints necessitate choices in where best to allocate scarce resources, our data suggest that a greater public health effect would be gained from widening access to ART for untreated patients with low CD4-cell counts who are at high risk of mortality rather than providing routine laboratory monitoring for people already receiving ART. (2010: 129)

Here, we are offered one rather particular interpretation of the findings to show 'what works', with the findings being taken out of the trial context and interpreted instead within the resource constraints of the policy context. In this case, what works is based not so much on the science, as on broader assumptions underwriting what it is feasible to do in resource-poor settings. Arguably, the issue is less about whether one or other method considered by the trial is better for the patients, but whether there is enough funding to deliver what is the best option. Furthermore in presenting what works, the DART study is not clear about what might be best for people who are already on ART who will in any case require monitoring through laboratory tests. It presents us with an interesting sequence of logic; in summary it suggests that we really like to save people and for that we will put them on ART, but once they are on ART we do not have enough resources for laboratory monitoring to maintain their quality of life.

This move from findings to a claim about what works provides interesting insight into the assumptions underwriting the analysis. One of the limitations that the authors report on is an interesting one when they say that, 'detailed analysis of viral load and resistance assays undertaken on stored specimens are in progress' (2010: 129). The fact that this is the case, however, does not stop them from concluding that

> …we have shown that routine laboratory monitoring for toxic effects in HIV patients receiving ART has no benefit. ART can be delivered safely with good quality clinical care, allowing treatment delivery to be decentralized. Small differences in disease progression suggest a role for CD4-cell testing from second year on ART to guide the switch to second-line ART. (2010: 130)

In other words, what is interpreted in the findings as 'what works' is only possible under the particular conditions of the trial, admitted to by the report, but which are not available outside of the trial context. This leads to a claim that uses the absence of trained staff to justify the relevance of the trial's results:

> …the interpretation of routine laboratory results by less well trained and supervised health-care workers with little access to diagnostic services and in-patient facilities would weaken the usefulness of the results and provide relatively less benefit than the small differences recorded. (2010: 129)

The assumption made here is not only about the usefulness of laboratory testing but also whether it is relevant or not in these settings, given that they are resource-poor. Implicit here are assumptions about resource allocation needs within the policy context. In this set of assumptions the choice is not considered in relation to long-term health outcomes. The idea is to use whatever limit resources available for increasing ART roll-out to save more lives. This approach does not taken into account what happens to those saved lives once they are on ARTs in the absence of resources for broader health needs. It is on this basis that the interpretation of the findings bets on CDM working better than LCM.

This position statement on what works is further justified in the *Lancet* report by the argument that 'irrespective of monitoring strategy, overall survival at 5 years was 88 %. The huge survival benefits from ART are well documented by historical comparison' (2010: 128). This claim engages the broader trope of 'saving lives' to underwrite the specific interpretation of what works by linking the findings of the trial to the fact that people on treatment have a better chance of survival. However, the fact that ART keeps more people alive is not what the trial was about, it was about what happens to those people who are kept alive when they are in receipt of ART over time. In addition, and on another level, the authors justify their findings and its relevance for policy on the basis of robustness provided by the high-follow-up and high retention rates over 6 years within the trial (2010: 128). While this claim may be relevant for the argument of 'what worked' within the specificities of the trial, there is nothing to suggest that the same thing would 'work' for health policy makers outside the trial and/or across Africa in general.

On the whole the policy position here that is based on 'what has worked' is related to how, under the experimental conditions of the trial, certain relations such as retention rates, the availability of high quality health professionals and the availability of laboratories to check if things were going wrong, produced the results that are now being interpreted. The main finding highlighted is the 'insignificant difference' between the LCM- and the CDM-based intervention for patient survival rates. But this in itself does not immediately suggest any one clear policy formulation. The missing link in the analysis is an explanation for the move from the research findings to what works. This requires attention to the differences between the experimental conditions and the real life contexts in which what worked in the study, must also need to work.

6.3 Possibility of Generalizability as Policy Transfers

In the previous section, I unpacked the relationship between particular research findings and the claim to what works that these represent for policy makers. The analysis suggests there can be a significant gap between research findings and later claims about effects and effectiveness. Policy based on the claim *it works here* may justify itself on the trial's findings. This conceals the fact that it remains unclear whether the findings would work as policy prescription outside the trial context itself. Any trial creates (indeed requires) its own special environment within which findings are generated. This context may differ substantially from the everyday settings in which even the trial participants live. By focusing more closely on these differences, this section will consider the next step in the policy process to claim that what works here, will also work for health policy-makers across Africa.

Even if one could for a moment assume that issue raised above concerning it worked here could be resolved within the context of a trial, a set of questions remain if the research findings are to be transformed into policy formulations in the form of *it works in general* and therefore *it will work for you*. These questions include (i) what was the procedure used to link the trial's findings on whether one way of intervening is inferior or not, to policy suggestions for Africa based on these findings; (ii) what was the procedure to follow in using this general advice as a policy guide in particular African contexts; (iii) is the qualification of 'good quality clinical care' in fact a *caveat emptor*[5]; and finally, (iv) considering that the trial was based on the full availability of medical resources independent of the resource limitations of the environment in which the study was conducted, is the presence of these resources relevant to the success of the policy as it might apply in general?

Underlying these questions of external validity (see Rol and Cartwright 2012: 191–92), are two areas of concern that play a central role in considering the ways in which research findings may be generalized from as policy advice. These concerns involve important assumptions about the environment and populations, and their interactions. Here, as in other instances, policy advice seeks to endorse the applicability of research findings across multiple sites. Although the DART trial itself was conducted in more than one site, the policy advice makes claims to relevance across Africa as a whole. The trial's findings were identified as a relationship between a particular environment and a particular group of participants. The way a given environment interacts with a population in relation to a given intervention tested in a trial, creates particular outcomes. Thus, the nature of these findings cannot be divorced from the particular interactions that took place within the trial. Because of this, a particular interaction between the environment, a population and the particular

[5]The concept is often described in law as '[A] warning that notifies a buyer that the goods he or she is buying are "as is", or subject to all defects'. Given the content of the policy and its delivery requirements and the way in which trial groups were monitored and participants' health was cared for, can this qualification really be a caveat or is it not, in fact, an *absolute necessity* for the policy to work?

intervention that is tested within the trial, frames the context of applicability of policies based on the given findings.

In a critical analysis of research methods on human behaviour and the way analysis usually considers the interaction between behaviour and the environment, Helen Longino highlights an important issue when she says that, 'the purported assumption that identifying correlates or even causes in particular environment is the same as identifying causes of traits *tout court*' (2013: 30). This is a caution that is also relevant to the present study. It cautions us not to assume that the interactions observed in one context can then be used to identify a general mechanism independent of their context of occurrence. Longino identifies two important issues here: the first, one of 'proscribing inferences from a single population to the species (or whatever larger grouping of population might be in question), and the second, [of] proscribing inferences in the other direction, from a population to its individual members' (2013: 30). When the applicability of the study findings to a larger African population is one of the central inferences drawn by the DART study, a further inference is made about the ability of health professionals to roll the intervention out on the basis of their abilities as observed under strict conditions within the trial context. Similarly, the availability of, and accessibility to, the resources needed for this policy intervention is assumed across all possible application contexts in Africa. Given the resource imbalances evident in most African health systems, and following Longino, it is not possible to infer that all environments within which the policy will be implemented are in any way identical (2013: 31).

There are number of ways of thinking about the environment in a trial and its implications for subsequent policy formulation. The circumstances in which a trial takes place create the environmental conditions in which the desired outcome is produced. For instance, the DART trial was run in four good quality medical centres in which medical staff were familiar with trial procedures in general and where there was access to required medical and human resources. Indeed, within the contexts in which they were located these centres were also centres of excellence in HIV care. Given the fact that the DART study was about the delivery of treatment, these conditions matter with respect to the findings of the trial. For policy purposes, it is essential to consider how any variation in these conditions might affect the outcomes if such an intervention is implemented in other contexts. A corollary to this must be a detailed analysis of parts of the environment that mattered most for the outcome produced. It is important to be clear about the fact that 'environments may vary over time and across space' and that assuming 'stability or variation in environments requires methods for independently identifying them' (Longino 2013: 30). These methodological considerations are not observable in the DART study or in the policy advice produced at the end of the trial. The population in this instance comprised the participants in the trial who were drawn from communities that had access to these health centres and who could be followed up regularly to generate the required data for the trial. Therefore, it is highly unlikely that participants in the trial were disease (or treatment) naive. The CDM intervention as a new way of delivering ARTwas operationalized within this environment, and with this group of people. A key question this raises relates to whether the way in which trial participants behaved here, can be generalized to others subject to these same interventions outside the trial. If the policy impetus is genuinely about the decentralization of ART delivery in rural Africa by delinking delivery from laboratory monitoring, the link between the trial environment and participants' behaviour within that context and in everyday contexts in rural Africa will have to be considered to be able to justify the policy.

This discussion of the environment, its interaction with participants, and its impact on the intervention can also be framed within the framework that Menno Rol and Cartwright call 'helping factors' (Rol and Cartwright 2012: 190). According to their view, right policy is rarely enough itself to produce desired outcomes. The key issue is the way in which within a trial findings are produced with the help of various contributing factors. Once a finding becomes a policy the availability of these helping factors will determine whether or not the policy will create the desired outcomes. Furthermore, they argue that success in obtaining desired policy outcomes will depend on the way in which these helping factors are distributed and relate to one another (or not) in the context of application (Rol and Cartwright 2012:192). According to this perspective, one can view the particular relationship between the environment and the population as helping factors to produce the findings of the DART study: the claimed insignificance of the differences between two interventions which then on cost grounds allows CDM to become the preferred intervention for policy advice in general. However, given that the intervention tested in the trial depends on the availability of HIV resources including treatment, health care specialists, the availability of next line drugs if needed, and patient compliance with follow up, the helping factors in this case are an essential prerequisite for the study findings themselves. In other words, the trial, by incorporating particular environmental conditions and people into its processes, created the very context in which its findings could emerge. The environment and the population are never auxiliary supports to an intervention but *underwrite the possibility of its success*, as the trial findings are contingent on presence of these factors.

This contingency raises questions about the way in which study findings can become generalizable policy advice. The link between the RCT as the context of the findings and subsequent policy advice with respect to implementation, relies on a set of methodological assumptions. It is not possible to argue that policy advice creates its own implementation context in the way that a trial does over time. In particular, the DART-based advice was framed within the assumption of an unavailability of resources, while the trial itself had had access to these resources. Longino argues that 'generalization beyond [that] population must assume similar population characteristics and similar environment' (2013: 28). The foundational assumption in this process is to assume that the environment of the trial is in some way analogous to the real life context within which the intervention will also work. For DART findings (or for the findings of any RCT) to have wider policy relevance, we must assume that 'environments other than the one in the study do not differ from it in causally significant ways' (Longino 2013:31). The justification for generalization assumes a mechanistic similarity between the way the intervention tested interacted with set of environmental conditions to produce the result, and how a similar intervention would interact with environmental conditions outside the trial. In the policy advice given following the DART trial, environmental conditions are taken to be homologues. Not paying attention to environmental conditions that may 'vary both individually and collectively' (Longino 2013:140) is a major concern.

The trial reports on findings from particular hospitals with particular resource infrastructures, including medical staff, where patients were monitored and evaluated according to strict procedures. A key question is how typical these hospitals are both in the countries where the trial took place, Uganda and Zimbabwe, and beyond in most of rural Africa? There is a further curious paradox here – the trial seeks to develop policy advice of relevance to rural Africa and yet the trial took place in a comparatively well-resourced hospital setting. Furthermore, if we assume that policy advice is an attempt to decentralize ART monitoring and delivery away from central hospitals, it seems to assume that the intervention will work independent of its environment. In considering a generalization from the trial an assumption about similarity in population characteristics will have to be considered together with the similarity of environmental conditions, a claim about biosocial commensurability. Given a difference in environmental conditions would the results still hold? How would people react to this intervention when they know about the lack of available resources? No real study or observations are available to analyze how in different medical centers/hospital under resource scarcity outside the trial ARV interventions and provision in general interact with people overtime and what kinds of health outcomes could be observed. Therefore, the policy prescription that is not considering these questions and only focusing on the fact that CDM worked in a trial is deficient. The policy would only be relevant if all contributing factors to create its desired outcome are addressed and available in each context.

These issues caution any easy generalization of the findings in a particular policy direction. Longino points out that 'if generalizations are to be obtained [from experimental studies]..., they will not be generalizations about populations, individuals or their properties but generalizations about processes' (2013:86). While this provides an interesting insight when thinking about questions of generalizability, in the case of the DART study it highlights one particular issue more directly. The DART trial was testing an intervention based on a process and the resulting policy advice was about changing the process of ART delivery. The trial was constructed to look at two ART delivery mechanisms, to assess similarity and differences between them in terms of health outcomes and cost effectiveness. In the process the main policy concern seems to be about choosing the most cost effective mechanism. In order to assess this, patients are closely followed up throughout the trial. Throughout the long observational frequency the difference between two mechanisms was assessed. While patients' participation and behavior in relation to the trial was important, the procedures created to run the trial were of more central importance. The trial created particular environmental conditions to maintain patient adherence overtime and the strict regulation of adherence, by medical follow ups by clinical staff, in the trial would have made a difference not only to the overall trial but also to the assessment of the observational part of it. In other words, the trial procedures, and the effect of the clinical trial apparatus itself may have contributed to the claimed non-inferiority outcome (Lock and Nguyen 2010: 185). However, will this be replicable in the absence of similar follow up procedures in real life contexts in rural Africa, and can the follow up and observation frequency procedures used in the trial be applied in rural Africa? Is, in fact, the claimed non-inferiority a *side-effect* of the trial process itself?

6.4 Conclusion

In this chapter, I have analyzed one case of policy advice within the Global AIDS system related to findings from one particular research study. The analysis has considered the way in which the RCT took place and how, in turn, its findings led to a more general advice to health policy-makers in Africa. It highlights major questions about the way in which RCT-based findings are transformed into policy formulations. Important questions were also raised concerning generalization from the findings of one trial to policy advice of supposed relevance to multi-site implementation. The analysis suggests that policy advice emanating from the DART study interprets the results of the trial in a way that assumes that causal variation in the everyday context of implementation does not matter with respect to achieving the desired outcomes. The manner in which trial results were translated into policy directions appears to de-socialize the ways in which people experience both HIV and interventions directed towards HIV in their own social and political environments. The social and economic dimensions of the intervention are considered only in relation to the technical aspects of the trial. This highlights important issues concerning the research knowledge-policy relationship both for AIDS in Africa, but also for Global AIDS in general.

The case study focused on here does not represent a unique situation in which RCT-based research is used as the justification for Africa-wide (or global) policy change. In the wealth of trial-based research that informs contemporary discussion of PreP, VMMC and other interventions, similar problems arise. In just about all the studies claiming real world relevance for interventions that have been found to be efficacious under carefully controlled conditions, it is suggested that the same treatment will be effective (i.e. will work to produce the same results) with similar populations.[6] According to Cartwright:

> To use RCT results as evidence for effectiveness we are generally told to look for populations or settings like those of the study. This is advice difficult to follow. We do RCTs because we do not know all the major relevant factors, so judging whether other situations are relevantly similar is hard. Moreover, similarity is rare. But then, similarity is not necessary if the treatment reliably promotes the outcome ... capacity claims provide evidence for

[6] In the case of VMMC debate, the discussion by Wamai et al. 2015 is interesting for its style of argument. Here, claims to effectiveness are based on the aggregate interpretation of all RCT and observational study results, when taken together. This leads the reader to assume some form of external validity, when in fact none has been demonstrated. This in turn is used to justify general policy prescriptions.

> effectiveness even in situations very different from those of any study. And where no capacity claims obtain, there is seldom warrant for assuming that a treatment that works somewhere will work anywhere else. (Cartwright 2011: 1401)

Neither the claim to have real world relevance nor claims about policy process in which one can assume the similarity of populations to project a capacity-for-effectiveness are straightforward interpretations. The assumptions underwriting these interpretations are often based on considering the similarity of the populations based on the categories that trials use, such as 'men who have sex with men', 'high risk gay men' and so on. And while these categories may be used to identify members of the broader populations that RCTs are supposed to relate to, there is nothing beyond these synthetic categories that will make these similarities relevant to the everyday lives of the people who are brought together as populations/communities for RCT and policy formulation purposes. There is also nothing in individual RCTs that will allow valid forms of generalizations to be made. As Cartwright further points out,

> [But] there are problems for using capacity claims. First, although knowledge that a treatment reliably promotes an outcome is evidence that it will cause that outcome for us, it is only part of an evidential argument. We also need to know that our situation contains all requisite helping factors and that there are no overwhelming countering causes. (Cartwright 2011: 1401)

This highlights that while RCTs may be able to make the claim that a treatment has worked within the limited context of a trial, there is nothing in this claim to suggest that a similar treatment will work outside the socio-political context within which the RCT was conducted, let alone in an entirely different socio-political context, without knowing what allows a particular treatment to become effective within the broader causal processes of everyday life. The possibility of interpreting RCTs results for policy development therefore requires knowledge that is not limited to the RCT itself.

The biomedical assumptions that underwrite RCT method do not provide good warrant for policy efficacy. This model, which is used most of the time to test the efficacy of a medicine in treating particular disease, assumes an overall level of commonality between study participants, their experiences of the disease, and the more general population in relation to that disease. A certain homology is assumed between participants in the trial and the populations they represent, in the way in which a pharmaceutical product might work. This, of course, is more questionable when RCTs are used to look at how social systems of resource delivery or access work (as in DART), as the 'treatment' here is in the form of specially constructed social arrangements for intervention that may be hard (if not impossible) to engineer in a similar way outside the trial itself.

Lock and Nguyen's view on this point is instructive. They point out that the biomedical approach 'works well in curing numerous acute, time-limited conditions that are essentially everywhere the same – broken bones, cataracts or acute infections – in which culture and environment play a relatively minor role when and how the condition manifests itself' (2010:186). Here, the claim to success is linked to the way in which the disease or the problem manifests itself. HIV and AIDS however are more complicated than basic infections or broken bones; they are 'conditions that exhibit significant variation in how they materialize and when they do so, tend to be chronic' (Lock and Nguyen 2010:186). Here, what we must look at is not just a bio-medically identified kind of disease kind that poses a particular health problem, but also the context within which the disease is experienced and the temporality of the way in which it becomes a health issue. Together, these factors locate the experience of disease within the context of everyday life. This poses challenges to the basic logic of RCTs, which aims to extract disease from everyday life, attempting to establish a causal relationship between a treatment and the condition in order to demonstrate the efficacy of the intervention that has taken place.

Given the policy-making culture in relation to global AIDS (Seckinelgin 2009a, b), policy interests have a multi-site focus. In many policy cases in AIDS discussions the assessment of efficacy cannot be isolated from the environment within which the study is done. As Longino argues, 'research cannot be separated from conceptions of what we want the resulting knowledge for' (2013:149). This then begs the question of highlighting who the 'we' is in the global AIDS system to provide the overall policy guidelines and the best practice guidelines for all of members of the AIDS community to follow.

I tend to agree with Lock and Nguyen when they describe experimental populations as 'contemporary "theaters of proof" where statistical technologies choreograph the performance' (2010: 202). My suspicion is that not only the populations, but the RCTs themselves have become theatres through which Global AIDS policy thinking is choreographed and performed with confidence. In this respect, the World Health Organization's 2015 Guidelines on PrEP are worth considering briefly. A WHO policy brief from November 2015 states that

> In 2014 WHO recommended offering PrEP to men who have sex with men (MSM). On the basis of further evidence of the effectiveness and acceptability of PrEP, WHO has now broadened the recommendation to include all population groups at substantial risk of HIV infection. Offering PrEP should be a priority for populations with an HIV incidence of about 3 per 100 person-years or higher. PrEP should be an additional prevention choice in a comprehensive package of services that also includes HIV testing, counselling, male and female condoms, lubricants, ARV treatment for partners with HIV infection, voluntary medical male circumcision and harm reduction interventions for people who use drugs. (2015: 1)

This is a most comprehensive endorsement of PrEP by the main international normative health organization. The statement is also comprehensive in terms of the populations it targets. It essentially makes all sexually active people in countries with generalized epidemics part of the population to be addressed. According to the policy brief, the key evidence for this approach comes from

> Twelve trials of the effectiveness of oral PrEP [that] have been conducted among serodiscordant couples, heterosexual men, women, MSM, people who inject drugs and transgender women. These trials took place in Africa, Asia, Europe, South America and the United States. (2015:1)

This globalizing narrative is intriguing in the way in which different populations are brought together as the categories listed with little attention given to the different experiences of people in the trials, or to their lives in different contexts. The issue here is settled on the basis of statistical evidence showing that PrEP as a pill delivered in particular manner worked for some of the individuals participating in '12 trials'. This last point is then used to merge the results of different trials into an interpretation that supports a single efficacious outcome.

Each trial was at some level trying to assess the efficacy of PrEP in preventing HIV infection. However, trials focused on different groups – serodiscordant-heterosexual couples, men-who-have-sex with men, injecting drug users, transgender people, and women in different socio-cultural contexts with different age differentiations. It is safe to assume that each trial revealed a different capacity claim in relation to the limited number of participants[7] included in the trial, with different trials giving rise to different capacity claims. Furthermore, each trial suggests that adherence is central to the capacity claims demonstrated, with adherence in every case being supported by the trial procedures themselves. But even under these conditions, the Fem-PrEP trial in Kenya, Tanzania and South Africa, for instance, covering 2120 women had to be stopped due to adherence problems among some participants.[8]

There are several problematic issues here. First, what are the implications of trials that had to be stopped due to adherence problems for interpreting the results of other trials? Second, how legitimately can we bring together the results from these 12 trials to provide general advice based on a overall capacity claim from the trials? Third, how do we generalize from this to the much wider populations targeted by the WHO guidelines, especially when the trials themselves were in specific socio-cultural contexts and based on the particular risk groups identified within these contexts? Finally, what is the best mechanism by which to combine the very different kinds of evidence elicited by these varied studies into an aggregate and generalizable

---

[7] The issue here is also about the number of people who participate in these individual trials. While the cumulative number of people participated in 12 trials may appear large, each trial had different numbers of participants. These range from 400 participants in the *Ipergay* trial in France and Canada, to 2499 participants across 11 study sites in 6 countries (the USA, Ecuador, South Africa, Peru, Brazil and Thailand) in *iPrEx*. The *Bangkok Tenofovir* Study included 2413 participants focusing on injecting drug users while Botswana *TDF2* study included 1219 sexually active male and female participants. There is the question here whether these numbers can simply be added together to create a total number of participants through which the efficacy of PrEP is demonstrated. Moreover, how individually or collectively do they relate to the larger population targeted by WHO guidelines? While one can imagine an argument that, for example, trial procedures create a commonality of adherence in support of a claim to global efficacy, this argument becomes redundant as such uniform adherence cannot be expected outside the trial context(s) as a longer-term outcome given the diversity of participants and their socio-cultural and political contexts.

[8] The FEM-PrEP clinical trial was designed to assess whether a daily dose of the antiretroviral Truvada is safe and effective in preventing HIV infection among women at high risk of HIV exposure. In this Phase III, randomized, placebo-controlled trial, 2120 women were assigned to receive either Truvada or a placebo containing no active drug for approximately 12 months and came in for monthly clinic visits for approximately 14 months (Fem-PrEP 2016).

whole? Given these questions, there are reasons to be seriously cautious about the policy-related conclusions that it seems legitimate to make.

This approach, which involves putting evidence from 12 trials together, has been widely used in other HIV-related policy manoeuvres – as justification for the mass medical circumcision of sexually active men in Africa, for example, where the results of three field trials were brought together to determine what must be done. It turns the RCT-modality in general into the theatre of proof for AIDS policy and a space for the performance of Global AIDS. The relationship between the RCT logic and global AIDS policy needs facilitates the simplification of the message by reducing to banality the complexity of life experience in different contexts. The idea of targeting those who are most at risk (be they key populations or others) creates legitimacy for the view that we are dealing with broadly similar populations impacted on in similar ways by HIV and AIDS, as global risk categories. This is at best an over-simplification and at worst a serious misconstrual of the everyday lives in context.

Chapter 7
Context Matters! But Why?

The importance of context has grown for me as I have participated in research discussions at conferences where new medical discoveries on HIV have been presented. These have included discussions on new ways of delivering medications, the effects of new treatment drugs, and even different ways of influencing sexual practices and behaviour change. What is striking at many of these events are the last few moments of the scientific presentation. Here, presenters typically report on the efficacy of new interventions or treatments, or on the generalization of medical procedures to larger populations such as has taken place with respect to voluntary medical male circumcision as an intervention to reduce HIV transmission. In these last moments of the talk, the audience is typically reminded of the novelty of the approach, the efficaciousness of the method of intervention, and the importance of this approach for tackling HIV, often with a statement to the effect that it is provides 'the latest weapon in our arsenal'. The speaker sometimes offers a brief caveat that adherence and context of course matter for the right outcomes, and then stops the presentation to take questions.

The euphoria attached to such presentations often obscures the caveat however. Most listeners conclude positively that we now have a new approach to reducing the likelihood of HIV infection, or influencing the behaviour of those who are at risk, or a new compound to deal with the disease independent of behaviour. The way forward for many audience members at that moment, and often afterwards, is how to get this or that new efficacious method of intervention to become part of the global policy processes and implementation. The policy relevance of a new intervention is inferred from the evidence of novelty and efficacy presented. But what about the short caveat nearly uttered and the question of context? If it is true that context really does matter, then what does this mean for the presented new approach and its policy relevance? And what does it mean also for the drive to make this knowledge immediately available as the basis for policy implementation and in many countries and communities?

In 2010, in one memorable conference session, while talking to an audience of over two thousand people, one commentator stated that the idea of 'treatment as

H. Seckinelgin, *The Politics of Global AIDS*, Social Aspects of HIV 3,
DOI 10.1007/978-3-319-46013-0_7

prevention' was ground breaking, and went on to say that as the research presented at that conference had shown, with treatment as prevention 'we don't even have to use condoms anymore'. His interest lay in interpreting the policy implications of one of the central discussions at the conference, namely the role that treatment drugs might play as a means of preventing HIV transmission. Arguably, he was generalizing from the research findings presented without taking into account caveats about context. Given the power of this mode of address, is it enough to add on as a disclaimer that context matters? If context really does matter, is it not the responsibility of the researcher presenting the paper to explicitly and in a detailed way show *how* it matters for a particular study and the knowledge claim made, and how this helps others to understand the research? Moreover, if context really matters, it is so because it was instrumental to the production of the particular results that have been presented. It follows that generalized presentations of efficacy such as, that medical male circumcision impacts on infection rates, or PrEP protects against HIV infection, should be presented in a way that shows under what conditions the results were produced, and in what kind of policy contexts findings may have policy relevance.

The previous chapter highlighted that while experimental methods, and in particular Randomized Controlled Trials (RCTs), have become the preferred option for policy design within the global governance of AIDS, there are important questions to be answered in relation to the implementation of the knowledge that has been obtained on the basis of these methods, across diverse socio-political and cultural contexts. This issue is well recognized as the problem of external validity in methodological discussions of RCTs (Cartwright and Hardie 2012: 45–46). Despite this, as an experimental approach, RCTs remain the preferred evidence source for medically-driven policy making at the global level. Using the knowledge developed through RCTs, global policy actors such as WHO and UNAIDS as well as civil society groups create policy guidelines and best practice examples to be used as part of global interventions to tackle HIV. This preference conflates knowledge production with policy justification. Moreover, this approach to knowledge utilisation, whereby the policy process becomes the means of generalizing research findings, has structural limits. While experimental knowledge production may be regulated according to strict scientific conventions, considerations of 'context' with respect to research findings and policy relevance is often addressed in a far more cavalier way.

In response, some medical scientists counter argue that the move from knowledge as policy is a matter for policy makers, and that they simply report the results of their trials in a self-limiting way with suitable caveats at the end. But does this defence have more than rhetorical value given that most policy-relevant research in this field is now conducted as trials to see whether particular biomedical tools work, or not, as policy ideas? In order to engage with this question, I want to consider what is meant by context in this process of knowledge production and the implementation of policy based on the knowledge produced within the Global AIDS field.

7.1 Context

The Oxford English Dictionary defines context as 'the circumstances that form the setting for an event, statement, or idea, and in terms of which it can be fully understood'. There is also a definition from linguistic theory, which defines context as the textual relations, utterances and cognitive resources which make a given text comprehensible. Both of these definitions suggest the active construction of meaning within a set of relations that are imminent in everyday life. Beyond dictionary definitions of the concept, there are other sources that provide insight into how to think about context as an epistemological lens through which to understand everyday life. In this section, I will consider some of these ideas. The aim is to find a way of thinking more carefully about the caveat that context matters and to highlight the ambiguity of this statement in terms of how it is often added on at the end of scientific presentations.

In his approach to anthropology and reflections on culture, Clifford Geertz offers some important insights into how to think about context. Reflecting on culture, he argues that the concept is a semiotic one

> '[B]elieving, with Max Weber, that man is an animal suspended in webs of significance he himself spun, I take culture to be those webs, and the analysis of it to be therefore not an experimental science in search of law but an interpretive one in search of meaning' (1973: 5).

Such an approach might be seen as moving towards individualism, but Geertz immediately makes his position clear when he says that

> '[C]ulture, this acted document, thus is public, like a burlesqued wink…The thing to ask about a burlesqued wink…is not what their ontological status is. The thing to ask is what their import is: what it is, ridicule or challenge, irony or anger, snobbery or pride, that, in their occurrence and through their agency, is getting said' (1973: 10).

This approach locates meaning and meaning making with relational processes of knowing, understanding and acting – within a particular public. Geertz argues first that '[C]ulture is public because meaning is. You can't wink (or burlesque one) without knowing what counts as winking or how, physically to contract your eyelids' (1973: 12). But he then cautions that there is more to knowing what winking is, than just knowing how to wink. He focuses on the process beyond the observed physicality of winking to think about culture. He argues that

> 'culture consists of socially established structures of meaning in terms of which people do such things as signal of conspiracies and join them or perceive insults and answer them, is no more to say that it is a psychological phenomenon, a characteristic of someone's mind, personality, cognitive structure or whatever, than to say that Tantrism, genetics…the Common Law' (1973: 12–13).

Here, Geertz is presenting a position within which the behaviours of individuals are taken to be signs from which to read off the conditions that make that behaviour possible and, more importantly, meaningful to those who are interacting with each other. He points out that

> '[B]ehaviour must be attended to, and with some exactness, because it is through the flow of behaviour – or, more precisely, social action – that cultural forms find articulation. They find as well, of course, in various sorts of artefacts and various states of consciousness; but these draw their meaning from the role play (Wittgenstein would say their "use") in an ongoing pattern of life, not from any intrinsic relationships they bear to one another' (1973: 18).

The point here is about a dynamic culture that is made and remade by the way in which different forms of behaviour are used in social action. Thus, it is in behaving this way or that as a social action, that meanings rest and are re-worked within a particular set of interactions. While this is a dynamic process, it is not one that takes place in isolation, as meanings are meanings in relation to others and the other social actions related to these. Such a perspective is in line with Wittgenstein's position of language as use, which seems to have been one of the inspirations in Geertz's work when he writes

> '[C]ultural systems must have a minimal degree of coherence, else we would not call them systems' and emphasizes the fact that understanding 'what happens' is about interpreting 'what happens' in particular place, particular time to particular people and what they do (1973: 19).

Anthony Giddens' theory of structuration also provides a useful lens in thinking about context. In a seminal articulation, Giddens (1984) reflects on the relationship between structure and agency and how these cannot be articulated independent of each other. While agency maintains a degree of will to act within a given context and to influence the structures in which an individual is embedded, this embeddedness nonetheless also frames the possibilities of action and change. The social structure in other words provides resources, opportunities and constraints for action. What structuration theory allows us to see therefore is the relationship between agency and structure that provides the grounds of being and action for that agency over time. The idea that structure is not external to the individuals implies that individuals have an inherent relationship with structure. This relationship is arguably underwritten by the linguistic processes that ground thinking and memory for individuals within particular environments. Thus, the possibility of an individual's action is related to the interpretive possibilities of agency located within a structure, and in person's engagement with that structure. Moreover, agency is always already located within a particular relationship to structure through language and the way in which language frames cognitive possibilities.

Of relevance in this respect is Pierre Bourdieu's work on the concept of *habitus*. According to Bourdieu, social practice is influenced by *habitus* which he defines as 'embodied history, internalized as second nature .....' (1990: 56). His argument is that people's actions are based on the way their past is represented and internalized. This internalization also influences how people think about the future and what they do about it. For Bourdieu, class is an important determinant of how this or that past is internalized. The idea of *habitus* highlights that people's reactions, choices and actions in relations to events in their lives are always part of a larger cultural and social memory that is part of people. So, it is in their everyday practices of living that people reproduce particular ways of being and thinking. Bourdieu argues that 'practice emerges from the relationship between external constraints such as economic and socio-political conditions, and predispositions or unconscious internalizations of social constraints' (1990:50). These internalized social constraints, such as rules of behaviour or moral relations, are often expressed as forms of common sense. Geertz's view of common sense is helpful here when he argues that

> 'common sense can be taken as an illustration of a particular dominant institution. Common sense represents matters...as being what they are by the simple nature of the case. An air of "of-courseness" a sense of "it figures" is cast over things...They are depicted as being inherent in the situation, intrinsic aspects of the situation, the way things go' (1973: 139).

This view resonates with both Giddens' and Bourdieu's perspectives on internalized understandings of the past, structures, and how these inform social relations within a particular environment. The notion of common sense also implies a commonality of cognition within a particular setting and, as such, provides a good grounding to understand how people behave and how in this practice they relate to one another and thereby regulate their relations within a particular environment.

With these theories of social practice and society in mind, one can more explicitly develop a systems theory of society. Here I will briefly consider Goffman's work. In his 1959 book, *The Presentation of Self in Everyday Life*, he points out that

> '.... the self does not derive from its possessor, but from the whole scene of his action, being generated by that attribute of local events which renders them interpretable by witnesses. A correctly staged and witnesses scene leads the audience to impute a self to the performed character, but this imputation – this self – is a product of a scene that comes off, and is not a *cause* of it. The self then, as a performed character, is not an organic thing that has a particular location, whose fundamental fate is to be born, to mature and to die' (1961: 23–4).

What we can observe here is the self as the result of interaction between different selves and the principles of interaction these create. The self thereby acquires a social role within an interactive process. The process is at multiple levels of interaction creating both the self and the possibility of its social role within an institutional arrangement which carries, at the same time, the possibility of change resting on these interactions. Goffman articulates this position by arguing that

> The self...can be seen as something that resides in the arrangements prevailing in a social system for its members. The self in this sense is not a property of the person to whom it is attributed, but dwells rather in the pattern of social control that is exerted in connection with the person by himself and those around him. This kind of institutional arrangement does not so much support the self as constituted it (1961:168).

This articulation is further developed in his work on *Stigma* (1968). Here, he analyses the impacts of negative social relations on the creation of self, and how these lead to social pathologies in relation what is seen as common or normal in a particular environment. Goffman's argument is important because for him being in a society appears to mean that individuals are identified by the external attributes that make sense in that context. He argues that 'by personal identity, I have in mind... positive marks or identity pegs and the unique combination of life history items that comes to be attached to the individual with help of these pegs for his identity' (1968:74). This once again concerns the imputation of self that might be made in the light of relevant performances within a given context. It is through these performances that society locates the individual in a certain role and comprehends their belonging. As a result, the individual needs to regulate their self-appearance by controlling how she appears within a given normality or situation of 'common sense', as discussed above – in dealing with stigma for example.

This position appears akin to that of the social constructivist and while Goffman accepts this interpretation, he also distances himself from it when he says, '.... where I differ from social constructionist is that I don't think the individual himself or herself does much of the constructing. He [she] rather comes to a world, already in some sense or other, established' (Verhoeven 1993: 324). I read this as an argument that by being brought up within a society, a person becomes 'established' in the ways and everyday interactions of that society. The possibility of participation within society rests in this kind of establishment of a person (also as a self-perception) through the endowments provided by linguistics and general cognitive capacities.

This argument signals the importance of Ian Hacking's (1995) discussion of *looping-kinds*. Hacking argues that there is an information loop between the way in which people are perceived in a society (or within the particular knowledge systems whereby they are designated as individuals, perhaps as 'risk groups' in Global AIDS discourse), and the way in which these perceptions inform self-recognition and awareness. Through social interaction people develop an image of themselves on the basis of how their social attributes are perceived by others. This process can head in a number of directions, including normalization as a sorting mechanism that confirms common sense and divergence from it, and which then moves on to stigmatize and exclude those selves that do not fit in with common sense. Hacking's work however highlights another layer of interaction between people in terms of how people's interactions are productive for each other on the basis of broader social understandings and knowledge. The important issue here is the relationship between language and cognition and the way in which language, as a shared medium, carries forward categories into personal interactions to inform the construction of the self. Important in this respect is Elizabeth Anscombe's (1957) work, related to that of Wittgenstein, which articulates the relationship between language and action. She articulates the idea of action under description. This is of critical importance as it argues that for an actor to act in one way or another, and for that actor to choose between this way or that way of acting, these possibilities, and what they might mean, need to be cognitively available. One can observe here the mechanism that allows both Goffman's person to appear as established and the individual to be established, as Bourdieu suggests, with the endowment of a past history and cultural memory that provides the resources and constraints for acting this way or another. The availability of this possibility rests with the language available to the actor.

This brief discussion of language categories and their effects highlights the way in which the idea of context has emerged in the social sciences. It also points to the foundational nature of context for the study of human behaviour. Within discussions in anthropology, sociology, social psychology and philosophy we can find the analytical resources to comprehend what it means to consider HIV and AIDS 'within context'. The idea of context in this way provides a framework within which to understand the relationship between human beings, the manner in which they become socialized, and how processes of socialization create the environment within which they conduct their everyday lives. It also seeks to explain how, in turn, this environment (society if you will), impacts on self-understanding and socialization.

In her writing, Germaine Tillion (2000) outlines the relationship between life experiences and the mechanisms that make them possible as comprising 'three central processes of comprehension, imagining and becoming in society' (49). Human beings comprehend themselves in relation to their social environment and others within that environment to think about themselves and become a person, by acting as someone who is comprehensible to others within that environment. Thus, when we talk about context what is meant on the one hand is the availability of resources to facilitate and limit this process. These include norms, values, material resources and modalities of being and acting with a given social environment such that participation in everyday life is possible and through such participation context is maintained. On the other hand, the idea of context is not only about these resources and modalities, it is centrally about processes and the ways in which these interact with each other and with people, and how they allow the articulation and re-articulation of sociability. These processes, through language and norms of acceptability, inclusion and exclusion, shape everyday practices leading to the issues that frame stigmatization, marginalization and their reproduction over time within social relations and, in different ways, as social responses to newly emerging interactions within a society.

These interactions and their productive nature, both as positive and negative, underpin the ability to develop HIV-related policies to help people. As Geertz suggests, these processes and the way they are made possible within a given relationality can be observed in the way people behave and act. The idea of context here includes a dynamic interaction between people themselves and the processes that allow interaction to take place in the first place. Here, the basic mechanism of both interacting to comprehend oneself and then to act in a social environment, is a function of the linguistic engagement that creates the conditions for imaging a way of being and acting as that being. Language, as Wittgenstein, Anscombe and others would have it, is the central mechanism that facilitates the production and reproduction of the context of possible and meaningful action in which people dwell.

7.2 Why Does This Matter?

According to this idea of context, the oft repeated caveat indicating that context matters in HIV research and in policy discussions is inadequate if the aim of its use is to highlight understanding of the context debate. The ambiguous use of 'context matters' in this way suggests that context might matter and perhaps needs to be considered for implementation purposes. The approach considers the context as something of an 'add-on' consideration. The implicit claim here is that the integrity of the research presented stands alone on its scientific grounds and that context becomes only an issue once we move to consider policy implementation, focusing on particular target/risk groups and the way we can deliver to them what we know works. In this focus on target groups, or as it is framed in present-day Global AIDS discussion – key affected populations – the idea of context becomes focused on individuated target populations for HIV-related intervention and what it means to be HIV affected for these groups. In most statements about context, these considerations are referenced to AIDS-centric knowledge and a policy gaze that first locates people in a generic manner within the Global AIDS world. Context then only becomes relevant to be able to provide policy interventions for such people.[1] Here, the idea of context as discussed above is considered as an externality that needs to be considered, controlled and manipulated a part of general policies designed to deal with HIV-related disease.

This situation leads to number of problems that frame the relationship between knowledge and policy within Global AIDS. First, by presenting context as an externality to research, policy thinking is orientated towards controlling this so that the research outcomes observed can be made replicable within a generalized policy framework. In other words, the concern here about context is about how to control it, rather than asking what it means for the research output. Second, when context becomes an externality in this way, people lose their particularity and specificity. Most HIV-related related policy interventions homogenize the people they target under particular categories. This abstracts people from the everyday worlds in which they encounter HIV-related interventions. It also means that they are abstracted from the context within which they became a person or someone who acts within a given society. Third, this in turn creates a separation between the everyday contexts in which HIV and AIDS are encountered and experienced, and the Global AIDS context that targets people as part of key populations, risk groups or whatever.

I would like to return now to the interview given by Mitchell Warren at AIDS 2014b in Melbourne. The second part of the interview highlights how social concerns are incorporated into the discussion as determined broadly by a biomedical science perspective. The interviewer begins by highlighting the social issues relevant for the discussion:

I. Of course this conference adds also a lot of social implications, decriminalization issues, the laws that are really being inhibitors, for the lack of progress.

MW. The elegance of the science, you see some of the science here, elegance of the science is remarkable. Even if everything happened exactly right scientifically if we don't deal

[1] For instance Barry Adam recognizes major challenges in relation to this debate, pointing out that moving from the idea of the population to the individual carries interpretive risks: 'Accomplishing widespread viral undetectability, even in highly-resourced settings, then appears to pose major challenges.

Shifting perspective from the population level to that of people who must manage risk in their everyday lives brings quite another range of considerations into view' (2011:5).

with that fundamental reality of stigma, discrimination, criminalization we will never end the epidemic. That is one of the challenges independent of no matter how many pills we deliver for prevention and treatment, no matter how many circumcisions, no matter how many condoms, if we continue to see laws criminalizing homosexuality, if we continue to see laws criminalizing drug use and sex work, we will never end the epidemic. No biomedical intervention can overcome those areas.

I. If people don't have that initiative, take initiative, because they feel inhibited in revealing their status because of laws. They won't be there to take the treatments, all these wonderful things, we have made available.

Warren agrees with the interviewer's last statement and provides the example of how laws criminalizing homosexuality laws in many countries stop many people having access to PrEP, even though WHO guidelines recommend PrEP to be integrated into prevention strategies for people at risk. He adds that

MW. We have to be careful how ....not only stigma affecting individuals but stigma affects our interventions. Right now PrEP could get stigmatized as *oh that's gay thing*, PrEP cannot be stigmatized like that because PrEP could have impact and prevent infections across all populations.

We are at this interesting point. If I think this issue of ending the epidemic by 2030, you need, in my mind, at least three things: you need a target so we got that, you need kind of guidelines and policies to support that so at least the WHO is a good example we have guidelines on key populations but you got to have the actual resources and the environment in which to do that work. So, we have great science that tells us it is possible, we have target that gets people excited, we have policies that are coming from global normative agencies that tell us this is what could and should happen. But, if we don't resource that, and if we don't really develop implementation plan, we will live in a world decades to come where those documents from 2014 are on a bookshelf collecting dust. We are in an interesting point, do we have the collective ability, wisdom and political will to translate targets and guidelines into practice. I do think we do.

I. That includes charging, encouraging and energizing the local populations, advocates, activists to do that work. It is hard for us to come in and look like we are pushing them… They have to be almost self-energized. I think this conference does some of that (AIDS 2014b).

The discussion is clearly aware of social issues. The focus is on the relationship between certain social attitudes and legal procedures stopping Global AIDS (ie. *our*) HIV-related interventions that are scientifically proven. Social issues such as criminalization and stigma are considered obstacles to be tackled so that our technologies can be used by people. While they are indeed obstacles, it is not clear what can be done about them unless their sources can be understood. The categorical approach evident in the discussion homogenises social issues, diverting attention away from the causes of these issues in different places. The idea of context evident here implies focusing on individual categorical issues instead of viewing them as evidence of broader social, cultural and political interactions within a particular situation or environment.

Another way of engaging with the substance of this interview is to focus on the sense of solidarity that underwrites the position of both interviewee and interviewer. Both talk enthusiastically about how to help those who are most affected by the epidemic. However, this solidarity seems largely based on how to get key populations to have access to 'our' policy framings. There is little to show interest beyond people as risk populations and risk groups. Individuals and communities are engaging with as people using only the Global AIDS categories. This is also evident in the way the conversation is about *us* and *we*. The use of the plural pronoun is clarified by the interviewee in the third part of the discussion when he talks about how the IAS conferences are important for sustaining the global response to end the epidemic. He says that

> 'to me 2015 and 2016 are the… there is a test for *us as community, for policy makers, for funders, for scientist, and for advocates, if we screw* it up if we don't take advantage of Vancouver 2 next year and Durban 2 in 2016 we will have missed the opportunity and I actually think that we won't get to 2030' (AIDS 2014b, my emphasis).

Warren's argument then is to keep us, the AIDS community, on the same page through the conferences so that work is concentrated on ending the epidemic by 2030. The description of us here has little to do with people living in diverse contexts experiencing HIV. Instead, the approach to dealing with the disease that has become 'our' problem, that is the problem of the Global AIDS community, and those people who 'we' are targeting with our policies become part of this community by receiving our technologies. It is clear from what is being said that the only context that matters in this debate is the context of Global AIDS and its interest in the pursuit of particular policy directions. Scientists and others are not in the least bit interested in the contexts within which most people experience sickness and disease, including HIV-related intervention, as part of their everyday lives.

The other significant issue highlighted in the language of both interviewee and the interviewer, is the individualistic approach taken. Even though the categories of risk populations frame the discussion, the focus is on the ability of individuals to respond to 'our' policies, including energizing them to tackle some of the issues. This assumes a distinction between the individual and their everyday context in terms of the agency to act in certain ways. In this way 'context' becomes something to be countered to allow individuals to act in the expected rational manner according to Global AIDS policy assumptions. One important and interesting example of this situation can be observed in relation to Voluntary Medical Male Circumcision debate.

7.3 Voluntary Medical Male Circumcision

In 2007, WHO and UNAIDS began formally to promote male circumcision (MC) in the form of Voluntary Medical Male Circumcision (VMMC) to prevent/reduce the risk of HIV acquisition for men in heterosexual relations based on the findings from three RCTs conducted (Auvert et al. 2005; Bailey et al. 2007; Gray et al. 2007), which demonstrated a reduction of up to 60 % in infection rates (WHO 2007). The recommendation was initially cautious when it said, '[M]ale circumcision does not provide complete protection against HIV'. Noting that other prevention methods remain relevant, people 'must continue to use other forms of protection such as male and female condoms' (WHO 2007: 2). Since this announcement, VMMC as an HIV prevention strategy has been introduced in 14 Sub-Saharan African countries with the aim of strongly encouraging men to undergo the procedure (WHO 2015). As a means to achieving this policy move, WHO and UNAIDS transformed research findings into policy to capitalize on the efficaciousness observed in the experimental settings. The underlying assumption was that the efficacy capacity of VMMC for HIV prevention observed in the trials is also a capacity for outcomes in real life and that VMMC will effectively deliver the expected results once implemented as policy. Since then, most policy statements on this issue, such as a later WHO and UNAIDS statement (2007) and the PEPFAR guidelines (2012), have been underpinned and to a degree legitimated by the results of three RCT studies conducted in South Africa, Kenya and Uganda.

The question here is how far the results of these trials can be considered to warrant claims of generalized effectiveness outcomes. One constraint here is about the kind of causal claim a trial produces. Cartwright and Hardie have written,

> 'Causal principles employed through the biological, medical and social sciences are *ceteris paribus* principles. They hold only "other things being equal", or,… with other things being "normal", or "within the appropriate bounds"' (Cartwright and Hardie 2012: 24, 25–30).

Such a statement makes it clear that a trial requires its own controlled context. Therefore, the move to consider policy recommendations outside of trial settings needs robust argument when applying a policy in contexts that cannot be controlled in a similarly systematic way. In other words, the context of the trial does not automatically warrant its application to *all* contexts. The reasons for this are related to the fact that beyond any trial itself, trial-based 'effectiveness prediction' (Cartwright and Hardie 2012: 41) needs to be reconsidered according to the different conditions, the 'causal ecology' if you like, that prevails in everyday contexts.

The RCT trial results clearly show that a number of environmental conditions most certainly contributed to the efficaciousness of the male circumcision interventions – conditions which medical scientists themselves acknowledge as potentially difficult to replicate in real life contexts. They include hygienic conditions, sterilized instruments, the careful monitoring of 'sexual activity' during the wound healing period, the training of personnel, post-operative care services and the provision of counselling on broader prevention methods, such as condom use, all delivered as part of the MC intervention (Auvert et al. 2005: 1109–1121; Gray et al. 2007 665–666). In addition, in one study '[P]articipants were screened to exclude those who were HIV seropositive, who had symptomatic illnesses, or contraindications to surgery. In standard public-health settings, HIV testing might not always be practical or acceptable… The participants in this study had frequent contact with study staff…' As the authors note 'This level of contact, intense counselling, and medical care is unlikely to pertain in standard settings' (Bailey et al. 2007: 654–655).

All of these considerations are structural and intimately linked to the delivery of VMMC. They should orient policy makers to think very carefully closely about the implementation context and the need to make this as similar as possible to the trial setting in order to achieve similar effects. But, with respect to these contextual factors, later policy discussions have been largely silent and the claims made run well beyond the evidence. For instance, Wamai et al. (2015: 646) have written that 'MC is likely to foster protective behaviour change'. It is not clear what this might mean in a context where understandings of male circumcision may be quite different to that in the trials, and affect people's reactions to it (Parkhurst et al. 2015). This position seems to assume that once a policy becomes part of the wider social context, people's behaviour will automatically change in the desired manner and that the results will sustainable over time. The question that remains unanswered here is whether this is possible if the mechanisms of sociability within a particular social setting, and which influence the decisions and actions taken within that context, remain unaccounted for in policy thought.

Male circumcision as a procedure is not about sex, but its meanings are constructed within the context of sexuality and the sexual practices and desires that influence behaviours. Given that as an intervention, VMMC needs to work with and in these contexts, technical delivery, or the act of circumcision alone, cannot engage with these dynamics.[2] A relevant illustration of this concerns available knowledge on the effects of context on condom use. Independent of condom availability, condom use is very much a function of sexual preferences and desires that are contextually determined. It is far from clear that this kind of contextual knowledge – on the local cognitive process that frame people's engagement with their sexual lives – has ever been part of male circumcision effectiveness assumptions when this procedure was turned into generalized policy as part of Global AIDS.

In a robust defence of VMMC in response to de Camargo's et al. (2013) criticisms of it as a policy response, Wamai et al. (2015) claim that MC is a superior intervention compared to condom based-interventions, given that condom use in similar contexts remains unsatisfactory. They argue that the criticism fails to take in to consideration:

> (1) a systematic review that included a trial, showing condom efficacy was 85 % for consistent use and (2) the lack of consistent condom use and demonstrated effectiveness in generalized HIV epidemics in SSA. Although the 100 % condom programme among sex workers in Thailand showed success, a recent Cochrane systematic review of the seven RCTs of condom found 'little clinical evidence of effectiveness' and no 'favourable results' for HIV. The reality is that, for various reasons, the use of condoms in both high and low prevalence settings remains at a level that is below that required to reach significant prevention thresholds at a population level and is declining in countries with high HIV prevalence such as Uganda, Cote d'Ivoire and South Africa (2015: 645–646).

The argument they offer here raises various questions. First, what does it mean to provide VMMC as an HIV prevention intervention in situations where condom use is low or declining, given that VMMC is never going to be 100 % protective on its

[2] Questions of gender relations and gendered attitudes towards sex (Connell 1995; Morell 2001) are important to consider here. Similarly, discussion of sex and sexuality in relation to health behaviour is central to understanding how particular outcomes may be brought about. There is also a need to take into account 'concern with "intersubjective" cultural meanings related to sexuality and their shared and collective qualities' (Corrêa et al. 2008: 133; see also Boyce 2012; Rohleder and Swartz 2012).

own? Second, with respect to risk compensation (for example, in the form of reduced levels of condom use), it is claimed that this was not observed in the three trials (Wamai et al. 2015: 646). However it is not clear how generalizable this RCT-based experience might be when translated via policy intervention into real-life implementation. Third, given that condom use concerns particular sexual practices, pleasures and desires, what is the relevance of these contextual issues to thinking about how these factors will interact with the expected effectiveness of VMMC? There seems good reason to expect that the real-life effectiveness of VMMC, just like condom use, will depend on these and other contextual influences.

So paradoxically, on the one hand we have here a dismissal of the real-life effectiveness of condom-use, itself known to be effective in trial-like situations, because of contextual factors. On the other hand, claims based on the findings of RCTs of VMMC are used to dismiss the importance of these same contextual factors. This seems to point to political factors influencing the claims observed in the policy-making process. Such approach turns male cuircumcision into a biomedical magic bullet, the 'latest in our arsenal'. In the words of (Wamai et al. 2015: 651), '[T]he world cannot afford the cost of inaction'. Such an argument uses prophetic language to trigger the emergency logic that makes the delivery of the technology the main concern. Contextual considerations concerning VMMC are most usually reduced to controlling sexual activity during the period immediately after the circumcision procedure by delaying sexual intercourse. The multi-layered complex contextual factors that VMMC requires in order to work within the everyday context of sex and desire, are downplayed or ignored.[3]

These debates on VMMC are directly related to the shared technocratic global AIDS thinking. The critical point here is about the influence of Global AIDS itself as a context for policy thought and how sociability within this system and the culture of research and policy practices 'impose[s] closure on problem framing and definition, the invention of alternatives, and the scope of costs and benefits [that] are considered' (Hoppe 2011:93).[4]

[3] Lack of interest in these issues is evident when Wamai et al. argue that the review by Weiss et al. (2010) 'noted there was "little evidence" of any adverse effect on sexual satisfaction or function following MC' (2015:643). The original statement in Weiss et al. concerned lack of evidence on the issue and did not reach a definitive conclusion about it (2010: S66–S67).

[4] This framing is much in evidence in a review article published by the *Lancet* to provide a state of the art analysis about the HIV infections at the time of AIDS 2014a, b, c in Melbourne. Gary Maartens, Connie Selum and Sharon R. Lewin list a number of breakthroughs in the abstract of the article, which 'include male medical circumcision, antiretrovirals to prevent mother-to-child transmission, antiretroviral therapy in people with HIV to prevent transmission, and antiretrovirals for pre-exposure prophylaxis' (2014: 258).

7.4 The Structural Drivers' Debate

Beyond the general awareness of social issues that can be observed in some aspects of policy formulation and debate, a number of social science approaches that have managed to influence the shaping of Global AIDS.[5] Here, I want to focus on just one of these – namely, the *structural drivers* framework – and the discussion it triggered. For the sake of brevity, I am not going to provide a full appraisal of the approach and its conceptual coherence. The approach does however pose a major challenge to dealing with HIV from a strictly biomedical lens.

Concern about the lack of structural analysis within the Global AIDS response was raised early on, as demonstrated in a special issue of the journal *AIDS* in 2000 devoted to the topic. In this issue, the papers included mirror broader discussion concerning the social determinants of health framework. For instance, in her introductory chapter, Esther Sumartojo states that 'HIV-related structural factors are defined as barriers to, or facilitators of, an individual's HIV-prevention behaviours. They directly or indirectly affect an individual's ability to avoid exposure to HIV' (2000: S3). She also argues that 'research on HIV prevention needs to target multiple levels, including individuals and environments that influence their behaviour. Biomedical and behavioural research has addressed HIV primarily at the level of individuals' (2000:S4).

This analysis, similar to other articles in the supplement, looks at the link between particular HIV prevention technologies such as condom use, and how certain structural issues act as barriers to effectiveness (Blankenship et al. 2000; Shriver et al. 2000 and Wohlfeiler 2000). There is a tension between trying to find a simple link between an intervention and clear structural barriers (a direct causality) and focusing on individuals and their behaviour as being personally motivated or exclusively resulting from a person's conscious decisions. This ignores 'the structural environment' and as a result many of these intervention are unable to address the causes of HIV risk.

A review article in the same supplement by Richard Parker, Delia Easton and Charles H. Klein considers how research 'has consistently focused on the interactive or synergistic effects of social factors such as poverty and economic exploitation, gender power, sexual oppression and racism in creating what can be described as forms of "structural violence", which directly determine the social vulnerability of groups and individuals' (2000: S23). This approach considers social structures as processes and practices within which people are located. Furthermore, it implicitly assumes that the ability of people to act, and their agency to do so, is formed within these processes. The authors observe that the 'systems in which diverse political processes and policies not only create the dynamic of the epidemic, [...] also

[5] One of these was the securitization debate linking insecurity to HIV transmission in conflict contexts. I have discussed this extensively elsewhere (Seckinelgin 2012a, 2009b). Another area is related to Catherine Campbell's work on 'HIV competent communities' (2013). I decided to focus here on the broader framework of *structural drivers* as this has become more widely termed in policy circles.

provide what is potentially the most effective source for intervention in order to curb its impact' (2000: S23).[6] The authors end their analysis by highlighting a number of questions for research and methodology and argue that the 'time has surely come to strike out in new directions that explicitly attempt to achieve more broad-based social structural change' (2000:S30).

More widely, the supplement's arguments reveal the form in which socio-political analysis at that time, and perhaps the social sciences more generally, was being incorporated into the Global AIDS system. The incorporation relied on public health frameworks and a focus on social determinants. As a result, the less predictable, more interactive and more nuanced aspects of debate were marginalized in favour of a focus on structural variables considered relevant to tackling HIV and AIDS.

The major, albeit basic, insight provided by the social sciences at that time was the fact that an individual's experiences of HIV and AIDS are subject to broader environmental influences that interact with and affect individual behaviour. This was recognized by the Global AIDS system, as shown both by the inclusion of structural drivers working group in the *aids 2031* initiative[7] and by the journal *AIDS*, which published a supplement on the topic in June 2012 just before the IAS AIDS 2012 conference in Washington DC. In their paper in this issue, Catherine Hankins and Barbara de Zalduondo provide a useful analysis that locates this process within the international system. They highlight how evaluations of longstanding individual behaviour-based prevention strategies revealed the need for a different approach by the early 2000s, which led to the development of the 'combination prevention' approach. While the term was first used in a speech given by Peter Piot, the then Executive Director of UNAIDS, during a speech at the 1998 Geneva International AIDS Conference, and an early definition of combination prevention emerged in 2003 in the work of Global HIV Prevention Working Group which broadened HIV prevention approach to include structural concerns, consensus on the definition and the need for combination prevention only emerged at the 2008 Mexico International AIDS conference (2010: S71–S72).[8] And while Hankins and de Zalduondo strongly support the inclusion of structural interventions within this approach, they also highlight a set of issues that make these difficult to use in policy making. These include a 'relatively thin evidence base', lack of clarity as to what amounts to a 'structural intervention', 'lack of clarity on the time required for effects and durations', and 'lack of operational guidance' (2010: S76). The authors recognize that no single conceptual framework can be sufficient given the diversity of social-structural issues that form part of the discussion on structural interventions. Yet, they talk significantly about the necessity of 'a common framework' to 'help build the global

[6] As an aside, this quote also makes an interesting observation about the impact of the Global AIDS system as a political and policy structure within which people are located.

[7] The aids2031 initiative was established in 2007 to review existing interventions and to signal future directions http://www.aids2031.org

[8] It is interesting to note how over this period prevention priorities competed with the question of treatment roll-out in resource poor settings as a global policy priority.

knowledge and evidence' (2010: S75). There are two ways of thinking about this statement. Given the fact that both authors at that time were staff members of UNAIDS, and Hankins in particular was a senior member of staff, this is clearly a statement of UNAIDS and other policy actors' position concerning structural interventions. It is also a significant advocacy statement providing guidance for researchers and others on how to influence policy makers if they want this approach to be engaged with as part of in Global AIDS discussion.

The impact of the orientation towards the social sciences highlighted by Hankins and Zalduondo can be observed in a subsequent supplement to the journal *Global Public Health*, edited to include discussions from the aids 2031 Structural Drivers Working group which aimed to understand 'the key political, social and economic "drivers" or determinants of HIV and AIDS' (Ogden et al. 2011a: S286). In this articulation of the structural drivers concept, there is foundational interest in the idea of context as discussed above. There is also a clear shift towards considering structural drivers from the perspective of the policy interests inherent in the Global AIDS approach. This is perhaps driven by the need to have an agency for change within the Global AIDS system. In other words, in order to keep policy actors' attention, the language of usefulness and operational possibilities for the existing Global AIDS policy thrust dominates the approach.

The key significant change here lies in the focus given to 'reducing vulnerability, rather than individual risk' (Ogden et al. 2011a: S286). The editors add that 'appropriately applied structural approaches create the conditions in which people can make healthy choices' (Ogden et al. 2011a: S286). However, they do not focus on what is meant by a healthy choice and who (or what) might provide the conditions for them beyond implicitly suggesting that these choices are in relation to policies developed at the global level. It is already clear that discussion here is trying to balance a view of HIV in context with the need to influence change within these contexts to so as to enable people with in them to exercise the rational choice to engage with Global AIDS policies. Each contribution in the supplement recognizes the complexity of social structures and identifies aspects of it that are relevant to consider. But, then, when discussion turns to operational issues, there is a shift to considering structural relations only through the particular drivers that Global AIDS has identified.[9] Significantly, these selected drivers gradually become the place-holders for variables. These then become the general variables to use in considerations of key structures affecting women, youth, MSM or other policy target groups across

[9] This is observable in the following statement: '[T]hree approaches and case studies are considered in this paper: (1) Increasing the economic status of women (parts of sub-Saharan Africa); (2) Addressing violence against women (South Africa); and (3) Changing harmful gender norms (Latin America, south-east Asia).

While programmes addressing these factors have succeeded in reducing vulnerability in some settings, these successes are necessarily context-specific, and likely to have resulted from a more complex interplay of factors than might be apparent from the summaries presented below (Rao Gupta et al. 2011: S372).

different contexts (Chandler 2011; Rao Gupta et al. 2011; Baral 2011).[10] The richness of structural relations is thereby reduced to already observed or observable relations that will facilitate the implementation of Global AIDS policy. The general thrust of this relationship can be observed in the following statement, '[P]ublic health efforts aiming to intervene structurally must be locally informed and target *aspects of poverty* that are *relevant*' (Auerbach et al. 2011: S296 my emphasis). The idea of using *relevant* aspects of poverty is ambiguous as it is not clear who will decide what is relevant. While in theory such an approach might make sense, given that knowledge practices are already located within a Global AIDS approach this creates number of challenges. For example, is a commitment to being 'locally informed' good enough to ensure policy thinking is located within local structural dynamics? Furthermore, given that most policies are developed globally and in a decontextualized way, could the relevance requirement of public health interventions here be about picking and choosing structural aspects depending on expert view on what is really relevant to global policy concerns?

In their article in this same issue of *Global Public Health*, Judith Auerbach, Justin Parkhurst and Carlos Cáceres attempt to theoretically locate this approach by offering an interactionist account of how social structures and people are connected through the way in which behaviours are produced in everyday contexts. They differentiate their approach from the structural determinants approach used by UNAIDS[11] because they see the latter presenting 'definitional and measurement challenges' (2011: S294). They suggest using social drivers as a concept comprising the 'core social processes and arrangements' that are reflective of social and cultural norms, values, networks, structures and institutions that operate in concert with individuals' behaviours and practices to influence HIV epidemics in particular settings (2011: S295 my emphasis). The authors argue that what is required is a multi-layered approach to causality:

> ….. various factors contribute to disease are often non-linear, and a certain few of them can modify (i.e., increase or decrease) the effect of others (for example, economic migration might increase the effect of poverty on sexual risk, or provide a conduit through which poverty manifests in risk behaviour). What is critical to keep in mind, however, is that the effect of each contributing causal factor is often not independent of others: the risk parameter (or the amount to which it contributes positively or negatively to disease occurrence) may change depending on other mediating factors and the context in which it is seen' (2011:S296).

[10] For instance, the important point is made that 'Gender norms particularly for men also commonly promote, or at least condone, 'homophobia', or antihomosexuality. Evidence indicates, however, that programmes to address unequal gender norms among young men can reduce HIV vulnerability and enhance AIDS resilience by increasing respect for women, reducing the numbers of sexual' (Rao Gupta et al. 2011: S374). However, given lack of detailed contextual knowledge concerning the production and reproduction of gender norms, such recognition may only lead to general gender empowerment interventions without addressing the dynamics of the production of particular norms (see Seckinelgin 2012a, b).

[11] This addresses the 'social and structural factors, such as poverty, gender inequality, and human rights violations, that are not easily measured that increase people's vulnerability to HIV infection' (UNAIDS 2007).

This is about the context of HIV as providing the ground on which interventions can be developed within a given context. Auerbach, Parkhurst and Cáceres also acknowledge a number of foundational problems. These include the complexity of introducing their new approach within existing biomedical understanding; 'deciding where and how to frame social drivers and at which level to intervene' (2011: S306); and the need for a language shift in 'discussing how, in what circumstances, and for whom particular combinations of factors contribute to HIV vulnerability (or, conversely, resilience)' (2011: S306).

In order to overcome some of these problems, they put forward the idea of 'sociological plausibility' as a way of developing interventions that 'hypothesise causal links between social drivers and HIV vulnerability where such associations "make sociological sense", that is, where they are consistent with what is known about psychological, social, cultural, economic and political data in specific contexts' (2011: S297). This will be based on 'extant social science and epidemiological data' (Auerbach et al. 2011: S305). Such an approach is inspired by a biomedical approach whereby 'the absence of mechanistic data but where an association "makes biological sense", meaning that it is consistent with what is known about biochemical, anatomical, or pathophysiological data or animal models…' is seen as valuable. Auerbach, Parkhurst and Cáceres suggest a similar notion of 'sociological plausibility' as a way of hypothesising the causal links between social drivers' (2011: S296).

This is an interesting move in terms of in its linguistic strategy. First, it aims to have purchase within the Global AIDS community by stressing affinity with the biomedical. This, however, means that assumptions underpinning the biomedical approach are also seen as relevant when drawing inferences from social science data. Considering that biomedical case meta-assumptions need to be made about human beings and their health to allow these kinds of inferences to be made, it is not clear what this would mean for any properly sociological analysis seeking to develop a 'persuasive story' from the available data. Second the use of 'drivers' as a concept implicitly gives the impression that it is possible to find key, or core, drivers that will be policy relevant in producing the particular effects expected of HIV-related interventions. Moreover, choosing core drivers so that policy makers can engage with this approach too readily turns these drivers into proxy indicators. Elsewhere, one of the same authors shows sensitivity to this problem when he writes that '[T]he language of "drivers" particularly appeals within the public health community, whose members are accustomed to looking for causal determinants of illness. A risk with this language is that it can lead to an oversimplified view of causality' (Parkhurst 2014: 3). Combined with this, the idea of core drivers and their selection for inclusion in a sociologically persuasive narrative is questionable if it becomes a general heuristic tool.[12] In the context of Global AIDS, the starting point in making choices and decisions about the parameters to think about a context does not begin from nowhere. There are already well established positions about what matters as core

[12] According to one academic expert, during a discussion with UNAIDS and other policy actors on structural drivers in Geneva, he was directly asked whether he could identify five drivers that would allow policy makers to understand the approach and allow them to develop their work.

concerns for HIV. These provide, à la Anscombe, 'descriptions for action' within the field or more usually sets of assumptions that link individual behaviour and perceived structural issues in a mono-causal manner so as to ground policy thinking. It is not clear how simply adding new social variables will make existing descriptions for action on these issues either more dynamic or contextual.

Another example of the positioning of the social drivers approach within the Global AIDS lens is evident in the following statement: '[T]he aim of the Social Drivers Group was to illustrate how HIV epidemics interact with social (cultural, political and economic) factors, and to advise policy-makers and planners on how to address these factors to achieve their HIV prevention, care and treatment objectives (Ogden et al. 2011a: S286). Here, it is clear that the idea of structural drivers quickly becomes a tool for achieving already-established HIV prevention, care and treatment objectives. Structural drivers are considered just an additional 'weapon in the arsenal' to fight the disease where the framework for a global approach has already been set broadly from within a biomedical framing of what really matters.

In this, I am observing a number of ways in which a reductionist or instrumentalist approach to thinking about the structural and the social aspects of AIDS has emerged. Broadly, social factors are seen as relevant because they interact with what AIDS policy actors consider to be efficacious in fighting the disease. Even if many discussions now mention structural determinants and make reference to social variables and social factors, understanding of these is instrumentally deployed to facilitate only those interventions that are seen as 'relevant'. Thus, social drivers are relevant to implementation purposes only if they are fully known about and can increase the effectiveness of AIDS related policy outcomes (Rao Gupta et al. 2008). Within such a logic, if it is possible to isolate certain structural drivers or factors, it should be possible to know why differences in response to interventions emerge in different communities or countries. Here, differential outcomes are considered in a limited way: as differences in already identified key drivers and how these interact with HIV while ignoring the fact that different engagements, such as initial responses to HIV or political leadership, are already located within broader interactive contexts (Baldwin 2005; Fox et al. 2011). Interactions are also sought between those variables identified as relevant drivers for HIV prevention-related outcomes, rather than considering how broader social interactions construct particular ways of being and acting which locate particular experiences of HIV.[13] In the end, we have here an Global AIDS-centred position that then engages with structural drivers, rather than looks at structural drivers first to understand how these locate HIV within peoples' experiences and practices.

In more recent writing, Justin Parkhurst has warned against the general use of the term 'structural drivers' as a place holder for in-depth social science analysis. He points out that '[T]he language of drivers [..] risks downplaying the importance of

[13] An alternative approach to considering behaviour change and condom use can be seen in Kane Race's discussion of gay men's 'reflexive mediation between embodied habits and medical opinion'. This provides an example of how the analysis can be turned around to look at practices which take into account experiences of AIDS with context (2003: 377).

human agency, and the fact that within any structural environment, communities of individuals will construct their own sets of practices' (2014:3). This warning against treating people as the passive recipients of policies is relevant. Within the Global AIDS approach, this way of considering people as passive recipients allows talking about the social environment on the basis of already established key population targets and their social environments which are inhibiting their rational responses to *our* policies (see Auerbach 2009). This typically instrumental understanding of structural drivers falls short of conceptualizing these from within the idea of the context that produces and reproduces conditions of being, acting and sociability within a given social setting.[14] As a result, this approach misunderstands the constitutive role of context in how people understand themselves and act in certain ways. The interest does not seem to be on the analyses of deeper interactive relations between being and acting, and the factors observed.

The structural drivers' approach and the policy orientation that emerges from it is therefore firmly within the Global AIDS system and is subject to its framing of HIV as a particular kind of a problem. Even, if it may appear as an innovative approach, it offers only a very limited engagement with the idea of the context as the grounds on which to think about the position of HIV in people's lives. Ultimately, within such an approach lives are made sense of only in terms of how they are understood from within the Global AIDS context and from its compartmentalized policy arenas. As a result, within the Global AIDS system 'there are remarkably few alternatives actually under debate' (Bosso 1994: 184). Via processes such as these, Global AIDS policy promotes its own understanding of 'context' organised around target groups and related issues rather than through policy options developed from the lived experiences of people who may, or may not, fit the need categorical distinctions established by 'key populations'.

7.5 Conclusion

The discussion above reveals something of the 'group-think' prevalent within the Global AIDS community. Knowledge production and its interpretation are broadly based on biomedical science modalities warranted by claims to generalizability, which in turn make them appropriate to all the contexts in which HIV is observed.

[14] In another example of this tendency, Seeley et al. in introducing a journal special issue highlight the importance of paying attention to the centrally of structural intervention in treatment as prevention. They conclude that '[A]lthough the focus of the papers is largely from east and southern Africa, the findings are unlikely to be unique to these regions, as issues of marginalization (and associated stigma) and economic and gender inequality are all too common globally, and apply also to other at risk populations, such as men who have sex with men and persons who inject drugs' (2012:1–3). Arguably, one set of social factors and particular ways of dealing with their implications are seen as sufficiently general from within the Global AIDS system to engage with different risk groups.

Policy prescriptions based on this kind of knowledge process reach conclusions based on predictions about policy outcomes that are not warranted on contextual grounds. When the claim is made that context matters, it is considered to matter only for fine-tuning implementation and not for justifying or establishing a claim about the knowledge underwriting the policy recommendation.[15] In this way, the logic of the Global AIDS system trumps the contexts in which different people live. By relying on an assumed broad-based solidarity and scientific claims, this disempowers people within their own context(s) to have agency for change.

Cartwright and Hardie argue that 'to warrant a claim is to justify it to be true… warranting a claim, any claim, means marshalling reasons for it so that it is transparent why you have the right to be confident that the claim is true. It follows that warrant requires a good argument' (2012:15). There are no good contextual arguments that show and warrant why the particular policies currently considered to be important such as, PrEP, DART-related policies, VMMC, or microfinance interventions for gender empowerment, should work in different contexts. The context of the policy process within the Global AIDS system overrides the context of the everyday life of people affected by and living with HIV and AIDS.

Decontextualized Global AIDS thinking has created a general image of the disease and of people with HIV and how they should be treated by their communities. This in turn has allowed people with HIV to make resource claims treatment and support. It is at this point that the image of the abstract person living with HIV becomes challenging because the claim to be supported is essentially a political claim to changing the resource allocation systems within a given country, and such a claim cannot be made or addressed unless it is located within the contextual social, cultural and political processes discussed above. Ellen E. Foley and Anne Hendrixson have pertinently observed in relation to the 2007 UNAIDS' global campaign *Know your Epidemic, Know your Response* that '[K]nowing your epidemic necessarily disrupts the notion of a global problem; there is […] a disjuncture [here] between international norms and infrastructure and local implementation' (2011: S319). This highlights not only the contradictory approach followed by global policy actors – in which contexts of knowing and response are split – but also shows the importance of the following questions. Who exactly are the people who need to know their epidemic? Who are the claimants here politically (beyond those who simply described as having HIV)? What does it mean for people to know their HIV status in this or that context? What does it mean for people living with HIV to have HIV in a context of meanings that regulate their lives and claim their rights in the same context? What are the local resource relations that can support needs emerging from particular experiences of the epidemic in that context?

---

[15] The concept of 'retrofitting' existing policy thinking to concerns with the social aspects of AIDS is also a relevant refection here (Richey 2008: 217–218). Another lens to consider this is how it turns people's lives into projects via processes of what Whyte et al. (2013: 143) have called 'projectification'.

The answers to these questions and other like them have serious implications for understanding and acting sustainably in ways that support people living with HIV in their everyday lives. Context matters most when the policy interest shifts from the emergency logic of Global AIDS interventions to sustaining life over time. This requires an approach to dealing with particular needs as embedded within particular contexts.

Chapter 8
Conclusion: Emergency, Sustainability and Success

This book began by considering how the international system understands and engages with the needs of those who are addressed by its policies. To do this it analysed the emergence of the politics of Global AIDS and the institutionalization of its political and policy practices over time. Two key questions motivating the analysis were: how best to think about the politics of the global AIDS response today, and what are the implications of this for a future that should more broadly be about the politics of sustainability of lives? These questions were motivated by the shifting focus from the emergency logic that first defined the politics of the global AIDS response towards a longer-term approach.

In terms of the structure of this book, Chap. 1 set out to provide a general overview of what constitutes the global AIDS system at present, to identify the concerns that drive the book. The following chapters developed an argument not only about how the Global AIDS system emerged to establish itself as a competent authority, but also about how it came to reproduce itself over time. In this respect, two central mechanisms were identified: first, solidarity claims concerning the international AIDS movement, and second distinctive performance and knowledge practices, which frame the horizons of what needs to be done. The interactive relationship between peak level international agencies and organisations and communities of people living with HIV, develops and legitimates the systemic approach to HIV that Global AIDS has adopted, together with its knowledge practices. The latter are important because they constitute the 'technical arsenal' for responding to the epidemic and supporting people across the globe. As Sidibé and Buse have recently written,

> ….. the AIDS response is underpinned by the principle that action should be data-driven, evidence-informed, and results-oriented. Gathering good data is challenging, but it is essential to measure progress, target resources, and discover and document what works in real time; it is also the keystone of transparency and accountability… We can and must continue to make our actions ever more evidence-informed. Data is a governance input and output: it drives what we do and shows what we have achieved (Sidibé and Buse 2013a:2148).

H. Seckinelgin, *The Politics of Global AIDS*, Social Aspects of HIV 3,
DOI 10.1007/978-3-319-46013-0_8

These and similar claims are subsequently used to legitimate the Global AIDS system as it grounds its resource demands from wider global publics. Together, the chapters in this book describe and analyse the relations between the structures, processes and actors that produce and reproduce the system. They also reveal how the agency to influence and to change policy directions is distributed within the system. In this concluding chapter, I extend these arguments further to argue that the idea of solidarity that underpinned the emergence of Global AIDS cannot sustain a system that increasingly needs to engage with a different set of circumstances, ones framed by questions of sustainability. I do this by paying particular attention to the success claims that are and have been made, and how these have come to dominate recent debates concerning the HIV epidemic internationally.

8.1 Global AIDS and Its Horizons

Earlier, I have argued that long-term considerations have rarely been part of Global AIDS thinking due to the sense of perpetual emergency that the system has projected. More recently, a major changes have been taking place in the global health field, motivated partly by finance but also by developments leading up to the development of the Sustainable Development Goals in 2015 and their reframing of issues connected to global health. Debate has also been motivated by a increasing recognition that

> … the challenge of a decade, highlighting the extent to which reforms and improvements in health systems must be thought about in ways that are perhaps less technical than fundamentally ethical and political, and reminding us that decision making about these issues (like meetings on global public health) too often take place far from the places and people that they are intended to serve (Fried et al. 2012: S1).

In thinking about overall global health governance and structures, it is hard to ignore the role played by Global AIDS interventions and the priority given to them over the last two decades (see The Lancet Commission 2013).[1] However, it is also clear that the exceptional attention given to AIDS as singular disease, both by the international system and by the MDGs is under challenge. As Woodling and colleagues put it,

> Awareness of the impact of the financial crisis and the waning political traction of AIDS as a priority issue vis-a-vis 'rising' health issue areas looms large… also evident is a response to some of the criticisms of the AIDS response, particularly the complaints over the select disease-focused nature of the MDGs, its short-term nature, the biomedical bias of current responses and the need to escape from silo-based discrete development interventions (Woodling et al. 2012: S155–56).

[1] On the 20th anniversary of the World Bank Report 1993, *Investing in Health*, an independent commission of 25 renowned economist and public health experts re-evaluated and proposed a new investment architecture for global health. The commission's report *Global Health 2035: A World Converging in a Generation* was published in *The Lancet* on December 2013.

This debate has also triggered responses from within the Global AIDS system, and more specifically from UNAIDS, as it tries to identify more clearly its role over the coming decades.[2] Importantly, UNAIDS own discourse stresses the centrality of maintaining a clear focus on HIV (Sidibé and Buse 2013a; Sidibé and Buse 2013b).[3] But such a stance has generated internal debate. Robin Gorna, for instance, powerfully argues that

> Realpolitik tells us that era of exceptionalism is past. Determinedly fighting for a stand-alone response to AIDS simply will not work in most contexts. Yet a stand-alone, fully resourced and ambitious response is worth fighting for in many countries, especially those that continue to face hyper-epidemics such as the southern African countries, where more than 25 % of the adult population continue to live with HIV (2014:111).

Gorna's argument poses a challenge to the way in which the Global AIDS system has developed and sought to be supported in its work. While recognizing what the system as it has become, she emphasizes the importance of maintaining a local perspective because people experience and live with HIV in often quite different ways, and in the hardest hit regions and countries an ambitious response is still required. In this concluding chapter, I want to examine this debate.

In particular, I want to argue that the structural conditions that created Global AIDS have created limited capacity for change within the system. While actions such as enhanced access to treatment drugs have radically changed people's experience of HIV, the Global AIDS system has shown itself largely indifferent to bringing about *sustainable* change in the different contexts in which it has worked. The challenge lies in ensuring how such a system can think about sustainability when its mechanisms were created to deal with an emergency. Can it do this? More importantly, the emergency logic of Global AIDS is not only simply a policy approach, it also constitutes the master narrative underpinning the international response to HIV, and regulates the kinds of knowledge production and interventions that are seen as acceptable. Through such a narrative, the system creates and maintains a zone of exceptionality, which in turn seeks to make all related practices and processes truly 'exceptional' (Huysmans 1995; Fassin and Pandolfi 2010). This process has created a 'therapeutic domination' that 'reduces social agents to human bodies', subject to policies driven by the exceptional circumstances of AIDS (McFalls 2010, pp. 322–323). So, the move towards long-term planning required by more recent global health debates should not be seen as a simple policy reorientation. It is about changing the horizons of the response from a perpetual present to the future. This may

[2] An early sign of this can be seen in Peter Piot's 2006 article in the *Lancet* which outlines reasons why the international system should maintain the exceptionality of AIDS as a core feature of international development. One of his arguments was about the potential disappearance of direct funding for the existing AIDS system and its work, if the new global system changes its focus. A similar concern has also been expressed by Ellen E. Foley and Anne Hendrixson (2011) in an article questioning the crisis model of policy making in this field.

[3] In a response to their interlocutors on their *Comment* piece in the *Lancet* special issue, Sidibé and Buse point out that 'The aim of our Comment was twofold: to advocate the inclusion of key AIDS governance innovations, principles, and practices in the post-2015 development agenda, and to ignite debate on the future of global health governance' (2013b:1018).

prove challenging given that the capacities present within the Global AIDS system are those of crisis management and not sustainable development.

There are other difficulties to be faced as well. While the Global AIDS system still demonstrates, both internally and externally, aspects of the solidarity that is so central to the politics of the response, the quality of participation, and the capacity to influence change has diminished over time, as highly professionalized solidarity claims and their performances have been reproduced within the system. As Gorna has remarked, there is indeed

> … a deep irony in the fact that the community groups and activists who drove the AIDS movement have now become junior players. Perhaps it was inevitable that civil society groups would exercise less influence given the amount of time and energy that many put into fighting for space and for significant structural changes (Gorna 2014: 105).

Such a perspective implies an institutionalization of global AIDS processes that has created distance not only from civil society activism but also from those whose needs are to be met, and whose rhetorical belonging to the system legitimates the existence of Global AIDS. Seen from this perspective, it is hard to see how civil society participation can still be considered one of the pillars of UNAIDS' success, as is so frequently articulated in official statements such as that which follows:

> [T]he participation of people living with HIV was crucial to the legitimacy of AIDS initiatives, and directly improved the acceptability and effectiveness of programmes. The same is true of civil society organisations that are hardwired into AIDS governance arrangements—from board membership to reporting mechanisms (Sidibé and Buse 2013a: 2148).

The challenge also highlights how civil society language has been instrumentalized so as to drive help towards people in an emergency, rather than establish a response based on political participation and on claims made on needs.

Furthermore, this performance of solidarity supports the unequal distribution of knowledge power within the system: between those who produce knowledge, and thus inform policy, and those who are subject to these policies as technical interventions in their lives. Ultimately, the Global AIDS system designates differentiated forms of agency through the social relations it establishes. Some actors are recognized for their ability to frame the problem, decide on priorities and produce policies in line with intervention strategies. The agency of other actors' is articulated in their capacity to implement, to receive and to use the technologies provided to them by the system. This then is a solidarity to receive rather than to voice the existence of differences in the form of different needs and different aspirations in the overall pursuit of wellbeing.[4]

[4]As in the politics described by Rancière (2010).

8.2 Temporality and Sustainability

The need to think about how the fullness of peoples' overall lives and wellbeing is intimately linked to the global politics of AIDS today. A forward looking response requires us to consider questions of ownership and sustainability. At present, within the global AIDS system sustainability is about maintaining existing interventions that aim to deal with the disease and the institutional arrangements that have produced them. In a more future oriented approach, sustainability needs to be about supporting and creating the processes that facilitate people achieving wellbeing in their everyday contexts.[5]

Ideally the first two of these are checked by the third because it establishes the obligation to think carefully about institutional arrangements and how policies are developed. However, this obligation can only be recognized and function as a check within the system if people's political agency is recognized beyond a general solidarity based on being passively included within it. To date, Global AIDS has very firmly remained focused on the first two of the above elements, as identified implicitly in Vinh-Kim Nguyen's description of the mode of thinking that underwrites the system.

> ….. the fact that tens of millions suffer from AIDS means that hundreds and thousands die every year. This supports the claim that AIDS is a public health emergency…and emphasizes the need to develop rapid and at times improvised measures to get drugs to people. Yet, HIV is a slow and chronic condition, which means that the benefits of antiretroviral therapy do not occur until after at least several months of treatment. Thus while the epidemic may be a political emergency, it is rarely an emergency in clinical terms (2010:103).

Nguyen's position above how Global AIDS approach to treatment[6] is based on a somewhat limited understanding of what it is that needs to be sustained. Delivery is seen as the main aim in an emergency, but what happens to people who are on treatment appears unclear in terms of the systems' interest. The difference between the politics of an emergency and the logic of sustainability it underwrites, and peoples' actual needs for wellbeing, creates a political complication because their time horizons of present and future are located in different registers.

The political formula that has emerged within Global AIDS discourse to motivate support for those with HIV across the world is based broadly on an *emergency-humanitarian, needs-resources, donor driven* logic. This logic is about the politics

[5] Even though the language of human rights and AIDS is used more and more as a means of channelling resources, it is unclear whether this approach will also allow people to politically engage and challenge the Global AIDS system. If they can, then what are the mechanisms for this, how can people participate in debates to influence change, and what are the implications of this for resource relations within the Global AIDS system?

[6] The wellbeing of people with HIV has always been a concern for many and in particular for the thousands of civil society activists who have engaged various political systems throughout 1980s, and 1990s. Nonetheless, the introduction of antiretroviral medication and its impact made the long-term wellbeing of HIV positive people in their everyday lives a major challenge for a global AIDS system that emerged out of this earlier activism and was based on the politics of emergency.

of charity, in which a powerful set of actors identify (less powerful) targets to support and the resources needed to help them. The approach locates people living with HIV as recipients rather than as active political participants who can claim their needs as these emerge based on their rights from within different political contexts, both locally and globally.[7] There is a major challenge here both to the relevance of the agency of particular global actors to influence change in the future and how an emergency logic has created a short-term temporality within the Global AIDS system (Ophir 2010; Redfield 2010). While making resources available is important, the system approaches this issue from its own timeline and perspective without taking into account the conditions under which peoples' lives can be supported in the longer term and in the context of their everyday lives.

8.3 Success

The temporality that frames Global AIDS encourages the international HIV movement to focus on particular issues. It also marshals different actors' work in a common direction. Thiscan be observed in the numerous campaigns generated from within the Global AIDS system. An early illustration of this can be seen, for example, in WHO's *3 by 5* campaign to bring 3 million people within the ARV treatment system by 2005 (Kim and Amman 2004). A more recent example is provided by the *90-90-90* approach promoted by UNAIDS in 2014 as part of a higher order strategy to end the epidemic by 2030.[8] This states that 'By 2020, 90% of all people living with HIV will know their HIV status. By 2020, 90% of all people with diagnosed HIV infection will receive sustained antiretroviral therapy. By 2020, 90% of all people receiving antiretroviral therapy will have viral suppression' (UNAIDS 2014).

Linked to this, it has also been claimed that '[E]nding the AIDS epidemic is more than a historic obligation to the 39 million people who have died of the disease' (UNAIDS 2014:1). The overall horizon set by this focus on 'ending the epidemic' relates closely to the policy imperative of treatment access. As the same document goes on to say, 'Although many strategies will be needed to close the book on the AIDS epidemic, one thing is certain. *It will be impossible to end the epidemic without bringing HIV treatment to all who need it.*' (UNAIDS 2014: 2, emphasis added). In each and every one of these cases, Global AIDS concerns frame policy practice within a finite emergency framework, therefore seeking to foreclose the future by becoming the dominant temporality within which AIDS is

[7] This kind of political agency provided the grounds from which, as I discussed earlier, 1980s AIDS activism emerged. That experience clearly demonstrates the need to consider people as political actors rather as being part of a global system that incorporates them due to their HIV status and then allocates resources to them as it sees it necessary for dealing with HIV.

[8] United Nations General Assembly High-Level Meeting on Ending AIDS, which took place from 8 to 10 June 2016 in New York.

experienced. Within this process the set aims and the set timeline create frameworks for thinking what success might be within the global AIDS system.

Classic examples of this foreclosure can be seen in terms of how success in treatment campaigns is often presented. On its webpage, The Global Fund to Fight AIDS, Tuberculosis and Malaria states that

> The Global Fund partnership supports programs that have saved more than 17 million lives since 2002. Current projections show that more than 2 million lives are being saved each year. If current trends hold, by the end of 2016 the Global Fund partnership will have supported countries in saving more than 22 million lives (2016).

The text goes on to say more specifically that 'There are 15 million people around the world on treatment for HIV, 8.1 million of them through programmes supported by the Global Fund' (The Global Fund 2016).

The issue here is not about the very real importance of treatment for people living with HIV. The numbers cited are significant. But presenting them as people and lives 'saved' because they have access to ARVs creates a problem. It locates lives as *saved* only within the targets achieved according to Global AIDS priorities. It says little if anything about what else might need to be available beyond treatment to save lives in the sense that people live lives that they actually want to live. There are several important issues here. First, in the latest forms of global AIDS discourse, sustainability is largely construed as an institutional concern; namely that of sustaining the Global AIDS system so that it can bring more people into treatment. Second, success as numbers is turned into something that is internally accounted for within the system as a function of its outputs. Third, what happens to people's lives beyond having access to ARVs as a policy output disappears, although they still continue to live (often in very difficult circumstances) with HIV. Finally, people's evaluations of their experiences of the Global AIDS system are excluded from relevance as a meaningful way of thinking about the system. Evaluations and considerations of success tie the future to past simply because they maintain the desirability of particular kind of policy thought.

Considered from this viewpoint, evaluations of success becomes a self-justifying process leading to institutional claims such as the following: 'Ending the AIDS epidemic will inspire broader global health and development efforts, demonstrating what can be achieved through global solidarity, evidence-based action and multisectoral partnerships' (UNAIDS 2014:2). This language reflects the new global health debate and seeks to maintain the centrality of AIDS as a global concern by setting up the Global AIDS system and its successes as an ideal example (see for instance Siphon 2013). While it is indeed important to learn from experience, success considered and presented as a broad measure of output delivered, say X million lives saved, lacks serious engagement with the long-term sustainability of the quality and nature of the lives of those who are still living with HIV.

Here, the question of *where are we going,* becomes important. The answer is often given from the perspective of the permanent present and the emergency mode of response that defines that present within the Global AIDS system. The question of future directions however challenges this definition. It encourages us to reflect on and evaluate policy choices, and the desirability of these choices for those people whose lives are incorporated into the system. The question of desirability here is, foundationally, a question of politics. It raises the questions of who a policy, or action, is desirable for and how the decision about what is desirable for future is established. Peter Piot has recently written that

> [J]ust as for the whole AIDS response, we need a long-term view on evaluation that suffers from inexcusable short-term myopia. As the spread of HIV is driven by complex behaviours and structural determinants, and the available interventions are less than perfect, the population level impact of even highly intensive programmes such as Avahan may take several years after they reach their maximal coverage (Piot 2010:1).

This observation concerns not a disembodied situation that we just observe out there. It raises an interesting question: namely, how is it that over such a long period of time the Global AIDS system has maintained an emergency approach to AIDS by promoting short-term evaluation measures that, in turn, have been used to further justify the Global AIDS approach. Partially the answer to this is about the way in which the emergency focus is instrumentalized to maintain the interest of general public and funders to support the international AIDS system. Furthermore, it concerns how this instrumental approach limited the evaluation of success within the global AIDS system to what organizations such as UNAIDS *do*. In this way, evaluations of success are limited to the organizational ability to get things done within the system. Questions as to why agencies do what they do, and how they do it, remain outside of these concerns. Looked at more encompassingly, the desirability of the direction of travel should be about how far the Global AIDS system[9] can address long-term differentiated and contextualized wellbeing needs that exist and emerge over time. Evaluation of this kind is about sustainability – in the form of how far policies engage with the voices of those whose lives they seek to address, and how far interventions build local capacities to influence change and initiate new ways for people to deal with HIV in their lives.

8.4 Success in the Public Eye

As discussion of the new post-MDG global health architecture was being debated in 2014, the international health community was hit by a major Ebola epidemic in western Africa. This triggered much public discussion, but one which took the global AIDS response as a measure of success in considering what the proper response should be to Ebola.

[9] Relevant considerations to do with the Global AIDS system include: who participates in what and how, how does categorical risk identification drive policy targets, what are the policy priorities that underwrite major resource allocation negotiations, and what are the system's primary funding relations?

In a series of articles, *The Economist* magazine on its December 13, 2014 issue engaged with the challenges faced by the international community in dealing with Ebola. The first piece on this issue was entitled 'Heal thyself':

> The WHO has faced wide criticism for its role in allowing Ebola, which has now killed 6300 people to rage out of control in west Africa. Some of it's unfair. The WHO's experts were not alone in relaxing their guard in May, when the outbreak appeared to recede. And although the world seemed to expect it to send an army of health workers to the African bush, the WHO has only experts and supplies at its disposal and it sent both quickly. But the world's 'directing and coordinating' health authority did little in either during the crisis. As Ebola spread, it dawdled, leaving overstretched aid groups to pick up the slack.
>
> This is symptomatic. Two decades ago it did a poor job of coping with AIDS, so the UN created its own agency to fight the disease. Too often WHO's policies are shaped by politics, rather than the best medical evidence. In recent years the Gates Foundation bankrolled an institute to gather health statistics and evaluate health policies which is now regarded as more authoritative (2014a: 15–18).

The article is an attempt to analyse the situation by focusing on the role of WHO in dealing with Ebola. The initial analysis provides a balanced view and locates WHO within its mandate to monitor and provide expertise in public health to member states. However, it then moves on to compare this to the situation with AIDS and the position of the WHO in the early 1980s, implicitly arguing that earlier problems within the organization led to the creation of UNAIDS as a disease-specific organization for dealing with the problem. An interesting point to note here is the claim that the WHO is 'shaped by politics' rather than evidence. It is important to remember that the genesis of UNAIDS was also intensely political. Here, however, the reader is provided with the impression that the mechanisms created to deal with AIDS were much more successful. One reason given for this success was the focus of the new organisation on medical evidence and, presumably, on the way that this evidence was subsequently used in policy interventions to deal with AIDS.

The next article in the magazine appears under the title of *World Health Organization: Too big to fail*. This piece more directly unpacks what the writer sees as the problem with WHO, through the comparison drawn with UNAIDS.

> Perched on a hill in Geneva above the city's cluster of international agencies, the modernist headquarters of the World Health Organizations (WHO) seems a manifestation of the organization's grand mission: to lead the world health. But nearby sits a stinging remainder of is shortcomings. Visitors to the WHO must first pass the headquarters of UNAIDS, which was set up separately after the widespread loss of faith in the WHO's ability to tackle the AIDS epidemic. Two decades after that failure, many health experts fear history is repeating itself. After an outbreak of Ebola was identified in West Africa in March, the WHO's response was slow, disorganized and lacking in leadership. In September Ban Ki-moon, the UN secretary-general set up an independent Ebola mission.
>
> Ebola exposed weakness in the WHO's ability to respond to disease out-breaks. But it also highlighted deeper problems with the WHO, involving funding, structure and staff. The squeeze has seen the WHO continue to spend on chronic diseases and primary health care – but slash its budget for responding to disease outbreaks by half. This may have seemed reasonable: year after year, chronic disease and poor health care are bigger killers. But a rapid response to Ebola would have been far cheaper in the long run than scrambling to catch up (2014b: 56–57).

This article directly compares WHO with UNAIDS. In so doing, it asserts the success of the latter over the former in such a way that the new agency becomes a permanent remainder of the WHO's failure to act. The implicit claim is that WHO found itself *once again* in a similar situation to AIDS, with Ebola. This is further evidenced by the creation of an Ebola-specific mission by the UN Secretary-General in 2014. The comparison between the two organizations is however underwritten by broader debate about the importance of disease-specific organizational structures in engaging with the circumstances created by AIDS and then Ebola. The possibility of making such a comparison rests on the assumption, an evaluation stated nearly as common sense, that UNAIDS has been successful in dealing with HIV. While the article recognizes the role of WHO in engaging with chronic diseases and poor health care, it implies that the organization lacks the agility, funds and staff that allowed UNAIDS to become effective organization.[10]

Without dwelling further on this comparison, it is important to unpack briefly what might be meant by the UNAIDS' success story. The content of this story is, as I mentioned before, intimately connected with stating the numbers of people 'saved' in the fight against HIV. In addition, while the role of UNAIDS itself is strongly emphasized within this account, it is also clear that success belongs to the broader context of the global AIDS system, which includes numerous international actors, civil society groups, researchers of all kinds and policy entrepreneurs from national governments and international organizations across the world. As indicated earlier, given the lack of knowledge and resources at the beginning of 1980s, and the way people in which had to confront the disease under those circumstances, we find ourselves in a different situation at present. HIV positive people, at least in some contexts, consider the disease as not the death sentence it was once. And, in many developing countries, more and more people have access to life-saving treatments as the UNAIDS numbers indicate, and new biomedical developments such as PrEP offer new possibilities for controlling transmission. As a result, it is hard not to consider the qualitative and quantitative change a success, and at that an impressive change. But what kind of success is this?

An article in the December 22, 2014 issue of the *New Yorker* magazine touched on a number of issues relevant to the question of success. The article is entitled *Can AIDS be Cured? What the battle's next stage will look like* and was written by Jerome Groopman. Groopman is a well-established professor of medicine with a chair at Harvard Medical School and a number of other appointments. He also has a respectable research record on cancer and HIV. The article provides an interesting set of insights from someone who has worked in the AIDS field since the early 1980s. He begins by reflecting on how in the winter of 1981 he first encountered someone with a condition that afterwards was named as HIV. His narrative shows how difficult the circumstances were at the time as no one knew what this new condition was, with most professionals trying to deal with the patients as well as they

[10] This analysis is rather curious, in the way in which the article considers WHO versus UNAIDS as if these organizations are set apart. WHO was a founding co-sponsor of UNAIDS and remains a part of UNAIDS.

could. He then recounts how the treatment strategies as well as the medicines that were used for treatment changed over time, and how this has been a constant process of learning.

One of the milestones in this story was undoubtedly the introduction of 'medications into a "cocktail" in mid-1990s, mirroring the way oncologists treated cancer' (2014: 80). Groopman talks about the impact of this change by considering the condition of one of his patients. According to him, the patient's health improved dramatically: 'less than a month after beginning treatment his fever fell, his infections disappeared, his energy returned and he started to gain weight. The HIV in his bloodstream plummeted to an undetectable level, where it has remained' (2014:80). According to the patient himself, who wrote later that 'I am probably more likely to be hit by a truck than to die of AIDS' (2014:80), this was not a unique experience. Many others had similar experiences particularly in the industrialized world at the time. Groopman then adds that 'in the past 5 years, not one of the dozens of HIV patients I've cared for has died of the disease' (2014:80). This is without doubt a remarkable situation. However, he then argues that

> there are still tremendous hurdles. Thirty-five million people in the world are living with the virus. In sub-Saharan Africa, where most new cases are reported, sixty-three per cent of those eligible for the drug regimen do not receive it; those who do often fail to receive it in full. In the United States, a year's worth of HAART costs as many thousands of dollars per patient and the long-term side effects can be debilitating (2014:80).

In this brief summary the author identifies a remarkable number of challenges that remain, even if one accepts that the change since the early 1980s has been very significant. Considering that most people with HIV are living in sub-Saharan Africa, the simple fact is that many HIV positive people who are eligible to receive treatment still have no access to it. The way Groopman frames his remarks provides a caution against ongoing discussion claims of unbridled success. However, he does not stop here, he also raises another set of issues which need to be part of any proper discussion of success.

He reports on a discussion with Steven Deeks, who is a professor of medicine in the School of Medicine at University of California San Francisco. Deek's work has been the long-term consequences of living with HIV. He argues that 'antiretroviral drugs are designed to block HIV replication and they do that quite well', but Groopman adds, 'But they don't enable many patients to recover fully. The immune system improves enough to prevent AIDS, but, because the virus persists, the immune system must mount a continuous low-level chronic response. That creates chronic inflammation, which injures tissues' (2014:81). He continues by saying that 'the inflammation is exacerbated by side effects of the medicines. Early treatments caused anemia, nerve damage, and lipodystrophy – the wasting of limbs and face, and the deposits of fat around the belly. Lipodystrophy is still a major problem'. (2014:81).

While I am not a medical scientist and this book provides a political and social science analysis, the implications of what is reported here are important. These observations indicate that treatment drug access is not the end point for a HIV positive patient, but that their health needs change. These changes have important implications for policy to address the needs of HIV positive people. Reporting on Deeks' work, the article talks about how many of the patients have 'high levels of cholesterol and triglyceride' and how 'these can lead to organ damage. One serious consequence is heart disease, which appears to be caused by inflammation of the artery walls' (2014:81). In addition, Deeks has also observed 'lung, liver and skin cancers in his patients' (2014:81). After discussing these issues with a patient who had experienced some of these ailments and the interventions to deal with them, Groopman reflects on the fact that this patient's 'state-of-the-art treatment costs almost a hundred thousand dollars a year', which is covered by his 'insurances and the State of California' (2014:81). Towards the end of the piece, the author points out that for Deeks also the question is how 'can the world find the resources to build a system to deliver, on a daily basis, antiretroviral drugs to some 30 million people, many in very poor regions' (2014:81).

This is a humbling and sombre question. The issue here is not limited to delivering treatment, which is a major challenge in itself, but is about how the world can maintain people's health once they are receiving treatment drugs. Both Groopman and Deeks as medical scientists seem to think that the answer is discouraging and therefore they focus on finding a cure. However, as the article further delves into the issue of a cure, it is clear that is not going to be a simple matter either. Deeks' and Groopman's reflections provide a cautionary framing from within which to think about discussions of success. Their questioning focuses debate on the sustainability of people's overall lives and health after they have been on treatment.

In sum, the health concerns of HIV positive people do not stop with having access to treatment. According to this analysis, after treatment people enter a different a stage of life where their health concerns need to be addressed by broader health systems. And while the nature of the problems discussed here are of medical kind, they are fundamentally linked to the products delivered to address certain needs, their delivery mechanisms and how far what is being delivered can be provided in a sustainable manner to support HIV positive peoples' wellbeing across the world. Groopman's earlier comments on access to treatment highlight aspects of the major policy problem of how to keep people both alive and *living well*. His narrative highlights the major challenges faced by people even after they have access to the treatment, and goes beyond basic survival to engage with the sustainability of lives. The concern to save life in an emergency, which so dominated the initial governance of the disease both at local and global levels, needs to be reconsidered. This emergency logic needs to give way to a new logic to sustain lives over longer periods of time in their everyday circumstances. It also calls for a change in the measures that can be used to assess success in the future.

8.5 Success of What?

> The AIDS response has been remarkably successful in transforming a deafening demand for inclusive policy processes and evidence-informed, rights-based programmes into tangible achievements measured in lives saved and dignity restored. The most visible manifestations of these achievements are the more than 4 million people presently on antiretroviral treatment and the tremendous advances in overcoming the stigma and discrimination faced by people who inject drugs, men who have sex with men, and sex workers and their clients (Sidibé and Buse 2009).

While targets to be achieved may initially be set as goals for the international HIV response, in time these targets become transmogrified to signify 'achievement' and thus 'success' against HIV, as suggested in the *Economist* article. Here, the Global AIDS system has used its emergency framing to set lives saved *now* as a *meta*-measure.

This establishes a pattern of Global AIDS policy behaviour that has a number of characteristics. First, particular evaluation frameworks come to regulate relations within Global AIDS policy. Following this, each actor participating in this policy arena needs to show how well they are doing within a particular policy framework and, ultimately, all are measured according to the *meta*-measure. Second, individual policy targets are by their nature set progressively. In each case, implementers have to show that more is done, policy actors thus have to show how they are contributing to the narrative of progressive achievement of saving more lives, which then becomes translated into 'targets achieved' by global actors such as UNAIDS. Then these narratives of achievements are used to engage with public policy to show success in *saving lives.* And finally, policy targets mostly take the form of policy performance, output measures. These are used to tell a story to indicate improvements in peoples' lives in relation to their HIV experience.

Through this kind of process, organizational accountability measures become equated with social outcome measures. In addition, saving lives as policy is implicitly defined according to the delivery of particular biotechnical policy products and people's access to them. Their actual lives and whether or not they are really saved remains hidden within the accounting process. So, if one sets out to test 1000 people in an area, and if this number or close to it is achieved, then this indicates a high level of success. The crux of the matter here is about the difference between the numbers reached as policy intervention outputs and the actual efficacy of policy outcomes in people's lives. The former provides the success stories of coverage, which are then taken to indicate success in terms of organizational ability to accomplish what one is set out to achieve. However, whether an achievement framed in this manner is a success in terms of addressing the actual problems of those living with HIV as part of people's everyday lives remains an open question.

The key issue both at present, and into the future, is the sustainability of the lives of people living with HIV in very different socio-political, cultural and economic structures. To assess this more adequately, evaluation needs to focus more fully on participation and the voices of disparate groups of people living with HIV in what are often very different socio-political contexts.

8.6 Where Are We Going? Thinking About Success in the Future

I want to argue that the future in this field should be driven by a much greater concern for the sustainability of wellbeing among people living with HIV in different contexts. The article by Groopman clearly suggests that this concern has been part of everyday life for quite some time in industrialized resource rich contexts, and that it is gradually becoming a central concern in resource poor settings. This concern for sustainability and the wellbeing of people living with HIV means that while HIV-specific success is important, the overall possibility of wellbeing can neither be reduced to policies targeting only HIV, nor can it be about the survival of the Global AIDS system itself.

In considering what needs to be achieved by forward looking HIV-related policy, more holistic thinking is required, because infected and affected lives are always part of broader socio-political and cultural systems. This requires the politics of Global AIDS to re-evaluate its focus, moving beyond a focus on the delivery of new policy products (in line with within particular organizational imperatives), to consider the effects of these for sustaining people's everyday wellbeing beyond the point of access. Here, new measures of success are required to evaluate policies with respect to whether they sustain people's wellbeing over time or not, and how well they enable people to voice their needs. How best do we articulate such an approach?

As I have discussed elsewhere (2012b), forward thinking in this area might profitably be inspired by Amartya Sen's work on capabilities theory. The analytic aspects of this approach are particularly helpful in articulating policies or evaluating existing policies. The idea of capabilities, at least in my interpretation, locates those who are at the receiving end of the policies as the central reference point for any evaluation. On the one hand, this allows for an evaluation of existing politics of AIDS based on the experience of those most affected by the epidemic. On the other hand, it encourages thinking about people's wellbeing as being the *meta*-measure of success. The changes described above in relation to global HIV interventions require the politics of Global AIDS to be more fully concerned with HIV positive people's everyday lives as they are lived in particular settings. This is required so that HIV positive people can once again be actively involved in ensuring how their needs are addressed, and so become (again) political subjects and actors rather than policy targets.

Sen's capabilities approach to policy thinking concerns welfare evaluations of how people fare in their everyday lives. This is important because it allows evaluations to be more than technical outcome measures decided upon according to externally perceived needs relevant to a target group or risk category. This latter approach only evaluates how *we* target this or that risk group, rather than what *our* policies mean to *their* overall wellbeing in a particular life. Taking capabilities seriously allows policy makers to think of persons as socially situated people beyond their membership of risk groups. I will briefly outline Sen's approach,[11] and highlight some of the ways in which may help reframe discussion of success.

Sen considers capability assessment in relation to '(1) wellbeing and (2) the freedom to pursue well-being' (1992: 39). He argues that the nature of wellbeing is related to the 'quality of [a] person's being' (1992: 39). This is a central orientation, as the idea of quality is not externally given. Wellbeing is the combination of what a person wants to do and whether they are able to pursue it or not. The freedom aspects to think and to choose are central to all wellbeing considerations: a person's quality of being is achieved by the choices she or he is able to make from sets of available capabilities or, in Sen's own words, 'functionings are constitutive of a person's being, and evaluation of well-being has to take the form of an assessment of these constituent elements' (1992: 39). The operationalization of such as approach is about the relationship between capabilities and functionings. It is about the ways of living people choose to have and are able to achieve. Thus, 'capability is a set of vectors of functionings, reflecting the person's freedom to lead one type of life or another' (Sen 1992: 40). Sen also states that that 'if the achieved functionings constitute a person's well-being, then the capability to achieve functionings will constitute a person's freedom – the real opportunities – to have wellbeing' (Sen 1992: 40).

It is possible to consider different HIV-related interventions from such a perspective. For instance, access to treatment drugs will contribute to the capability set of an individual and towards her wellbeing by keeping her alive. It will also provide support to other components of the capabilities she might have. The ability to make choices based on this will however depend on other components and their availability to her. This is, of course, based on the availability of choice in the first place. While availability and access to ARV treatment provides the choice to use them, it will not change overall wellbeing unless that choice can be used by persons, and used for as long as they need to. This is critical because this relationship between the provision of a choice and the ability to take that choice underwrites what it is that the Global AIDS system needs to evaluate: if our measure of success is just to survive, this leads to looking at how many people have access to treatment. This does not say, however, whether people are properly 'saved', to the extent that they will live the lives they would like to live. It also suggests that the claim that the 'system saved lives' needs to be qualified, as it is time and context dependent at the point of delivery. Sen's articulation allows socio-political analysis to consider how well a person's freedoms within a given context allow her to achieve wellbeing in the way she chooses to function, and in ways that are valued by her (see Alkire 2001: 6–7). In other words, his view takes into account a persons' own consideration of their well-being and the way in which this contributes (or not) to broader aggregate social well-being. A capabilities approach thereby allows us to think beyond the provision of primary goods or particular commodities to engage more fully and holistically with people's lives and the lives they wish to live. It considers that the provision of resources such as treatment drugs will not necessarily result in

[11] Sen's work initiated an in-depth debate and literature on capabilities which I am not going to rehearse here (Seckinelgin 2004).

wellbeing outcomes if these are not translated into capabilities. Sen recently argued that 'it does make a difference whether we look merely at the means of living rather than directly at the lives that people managed to have' (2010: 3cc).

As discussed in the last chapter, in 2014 WHO published guidelines that strongly recommend the use of PrEP as a part of a combined prevention strategy particularly targeting key populations. This is one area where one can raise the question of evaluation and success: how will any implementation be evaluated? The relevance and the context of the WHO guidelines is made clear by Carlos F Cáceres, Kevin O'Reilly, Kenneth Mayer and Rachel Baggaley in their introduction to a special supplement published in the journal *AIDS* in 2015. They argue that

> despite the now well recognized preventive effects of ART in suppressing HIV infectiousness in treated patients, HIV incidence remains unacceptably high. This is particularly true in subgroups of the general population in generalized epidemic settings (e.g. young women in Africa) and in key populations [KPs; e.g.men and transgender women (TW) who have sex with men, injection drug users and sex workers] in both concentrated and generalized epidemics (Cáceres et al. 2015:1).

This view explicitly acknowledges that there is a need to reconsider the prevention strategies that Global AIDS has used so far. If, after decades of intervention, there are still issues of reach and efficaciousness that need to be addressed by HIV prevention policies, then there is an urgent need to consider that it is not simply enough to simply make biomedical technologies such as PrEP more widely available.

There are a number of ways to think about this. Biomedical and scientific research shows that PrEP has an important role to play in relation to HIV prevention (Kebaabetswe et al. 2014; Wade Taylor et al. 2014; Molina et al. 2015; Buchbinder and Liu 2015). Many studies describe the efficaciousness of the particular regimen of pills used in a specific way in reducing the probability of acquiring HIV by particular populations. This same body of research also broadly agrees that treatment adherence is central to success. The main issue in such accounts is the availability of PrEP and then the correct use of the procedure, adherence, if the expected outcome is to be produced.[12] This framing can also be expressed as the *capability* provided by the availability of PrEP to those persons who to decide to use it, their *functioning*. The outcome of reduced rates of HIV infection can be only achieved if these two work together and, in particular, if people use PrEP consistently over time before they engage in HIV risk-related sexual behaviour. This frame of reference already moves discussion beyond access and availability questions.[13] As important

[12] Molina et al. point out that 'assessing adherence to sexual activity-dependent preexposure prophylaxis is challenging and represents another limitation of our study' (2015: 2244). The challenge here is about the way in which people consider sex and also their own sexual subjectivity in relation to a product, which evidently aims in some manner to regulate it. This will also be more complicated in certain contexts. It is further argued that 'MSM who are at risk for acquiring HIV who elect to use PrEP need prevention counselling strategies to teach them to take PrEP on a daily and consistent basis' (Wade Taylor et al. 2014:2).

[13] Hankins et al. provide a nuanced understanding of these functional relations '[D]ecision-makers considering the introduction of PrEP in their countries are faced with competing priorities and the need to address key economic, regulatory, distributive justice and access issues. Unless these pro-

as these are, in the end whether people chose to use a medication, and how they use it, will determine success in terms of the goals set by the Global AIDS system: ie. reduced rates of infection. But can we legitimately expect enhanced availability by itself to lead to widespread use and the population level behaviour change that will lead to an overall reduction in HIV infections?

An answer to this question, or at least an approximation of it, was given by Peter Aggleton at the 2014 World AIDS Conference in Melbourne, as a part of a panel discussion on PrEP and gay men's health. On the question of whether 'the idea of advent of PrEP is an ordinary or an extraordinary event'. He said that 'I suspect that in 10 years' time we will be here and will conclude that it is *useful to some people, in some contexts, some of the time*, that is, exactly the same as condoms and indeed as negotiated safety' (2014c my emphasis). This statement succinctly points out that much will depend on the context and the way in which people targeted by PrEP policies engage with it, and are able to turn it into functioning in different contexts.[14] Some may consider this a simply question of adherence, as identified in the reports of medical trials on the issue. However, what is being articulated here is not about adherence as assumed rational behaviour once one is provided with the resources. Aggleton's point is about exercising the freedom to use or not to use. This is exactly the kind of freedom advocated for within discussions of capability based on the kinds of lives people chose to live. To me, this is important point since it indicates that even if PrEP provision appears as a potential capability, its transformation to a functioning will depend at least in part on the personal evaluation of its relevance and potential. It also suggests that in the end any policy evaluation needs to take account of contextual factors and what motivates people to engage with a new (or old) prevention option rather than simply focusing on provision and access in attributing success. Ignoring this, and targeting adherence from a narrow lens is not going to engage with the kind of freedom that it is also necessary to evaluate in how individuals negotiate to act within their particular context.

This poses a major challenge to the Global AIDS system in its biomedical mode and in its consideration of advances such as PrEP. As argued by Judith Auerbach and Trevor Hoppe, discussions of pre-exposure prophylaxis (PrEP) to date have largely focused on two questions: is it clinically effective, and what are the structural and policy factors that impact its effectiveness when implemented?' (2015:1). As they rightly point out, the second question, interpreted as a functional relationship

cesses are informed by inputs relative to their own specific context, it will be difficult to realize the full potential of effective and acceptable PrEP implementation' (2015:5).

[14] For example, a study based in the US South presented in the 2015 Conference on Retroviruses and Opportunistic Infections (CRIO) in Seattle highlights how such interventions are implemented within existing social contexts and how these contextual factors impact outcomes: 'The investigators conclude that disparities at various steps in the PrEP care continuum, particularly access to health care, could lead to racial disparities in those achieving protection via PrEP' (Buchbinder and Liu 2015:18). Another similarly context sensitive analysis can be found in a report of a PrEP trial in Botswana. Although the authors articulate the issue as an 'adherence problem', their concerns highlight how adherence is about a dynamic interactive relationship between persons and their contexts (Kebaaetswee et al. 2015).

between a number of already identified factors that will establish the right delivery mechanisms, does not allow for an understanding of what really makes people chose certain things when regulating their sexual lives. Put together with Aggleton's formula, matters become even more complex. Once these functionally recognized basic structural relations are put into context, they may well influence people differently in deciding whether to use PrEP or not, even where the individuals concerned may be considered to fall within the same risk category.

This clearly pushes us to think about the capability-functioning relationship within a particular context if we are to be able to provide support over time to people to maintain their wellbeing. Whether PrEP will 'work' is dependent on the context(s) within which people make choices, and how these choices are supported by other resources, including the material, social, and psychological ones on which individuals rely. Sen's position therefore provides us with the evaluative means with which to influence change within the Global AIDS system. It brings together what at present appear to be evaluations based on systemic justifications of the ways in which knowledge and policy are produced on the supply side, and what people are able to do with the things supplied to them within the system. Instead, discussion should follow Sen's position that 'the means of satisfactory human living are not themselves the ends of good living' but are the 'means to other things' (2010: 234). Future evaluations should seek to offer a comprehensive view of the link between the provision of particular means (ART-related services, for example) and how these may prove instrumental in achieving a good life within particular contexts.

But it is time to reach some kind of conclusion. The central argument throughout this book has been that sustainability of wellbeing of people living with HIV is the most important challenge facing the Global AIDS system today. The existing Global AIDS system is not well-equipped to face this challenge and requires serious overhaul. In this respect, it is key for policy makers to recognize the structural limits of the system that has been created to deal with HIV. Furthermore, the limits of solidarity that has acted as the glue of the existing system need to be recognized. Without these considerations, the system cannot comprehend how to engage with newly emerging needs related with wellbeing in diverse contexts. Against numerous attempts to bring more social research and analysis to the fore, the Global AIDS system has persisted in understanding HIV as little more than an infection (albeit one with potentially catastrophic effects). It is time that HIV is approached from the perspective of people living with it as a part of their everyday lives. Even if infection rates are reduced, there will still be millions of people living with HIV and the sustainability of their wellbeing over time matters. At present, independent of past resistance, it is imperative to place the temporal, the contextual, the social and the political analysis at the centre of our thinking about HIV and HIV policy processes. If we fail to do so, we run the risk of following policy fashions that come and go without dealing with the challenges of the sustainability of wellbeing. The cost of this will accrue to people living with HIV in many different parts of the world. Dealing with HIV now requires the system to recognize (once again) the socio-political agency of people living with HIV to influence change, both within the everyday social contexts in which they live, and within the Global AIDS system itself.

Bibliography

Adam, B. D. (2011). Epistemic fault lines in biomedical and social approaches to HIV prevention. *Journal of International AIDS Society, 14*(Suppl. 2), S2.

Aggleton, P. (2007). "Just a snip"? A social history of male circumcision. *Reproductive Health Matters, 15*, 15–21.

Aggleton, P., & Campbell, C. (1999). Young people's sexual health: A framework for policy debate. *Canadian Journal of Human Sexuality, 8*, 249–262.

Aggleton, P., & Wood, K. (2003). *Promoting young people's sexual and reproductive health stigma, discrimination and human rights*. London: Institute of Education, University of London.

Aggleton, P., Davies, P., & Hart, G. (1997). *AIDS: Activism and alliances*. London: Taylor & Francis.

Aginam, O., & Harrington, J. (2013). Introduction. In O. Aginam, J. Harrington, & P. K. Yu (Eds.), *The global governance of HIV/AIDS: Intellectual property and access to essential medicines* (pp. 1–13). Cheltenham: Edward Elgar.

AIDS. (2012a). *Activists interrupt press conference at AIDS 2012*. https://www.youtube.com/watch?v=FB_1fQZ8Ydg. Accessed 12 Mar 2016.

AIDS. (2012b). *Secretary Clinton delivers remarks at the 2012 international AIDS conference*. https://www.youtube.com/watch?v=9bnVNd4G9Ks. Accessed 25 Feb 2016.

AIDS. (2012c). *International AIDS conference 2012, plenary: Dynamics of the epidemic in context*. https://www.youtube.com/watch?v=3ZBKcvyMRA4. Accessed 18 Dec 2015.

AIDS. (2012d). *Christopher Beyrer: Do we have the political will to implement the new science to turn the tide?* https://www.youtube.com/watch?v=Xgtba3QlWu4. Accessed 18 Dec 2015.

AIDS. (2014a). *Ambassador Birx shares highlights from AIDS 2014 and introduces PEPFAR dashboards*. https://www.youtube.com/watch?v=bEWv0H-wHkg. Accessed 4 Dec 2015.

AIDS. (2014b). *AIDS 2014: Mitchell Warren*. https://www.youtube.com/watch?v=GZJaH3ATTIw. Accessed 4 Dec 2015.

AIDS. (2014c). *Gay men's heath and PrEP: The new community voices of activism*. https://www.youtube.com/watch?v=IyeBpFbroFA. Accessed 5 Mar 2016.

AIDS. (2016a). *Conference committees*. http://www.aids2016.org/About/Committees. Accessed 26 Mar 2016.

AIDS. (2016b). *Abstract submission tutorial*. http://www.aids2016.org/Programme/Abstracts/Submission-Guidelines. Accessed 26 Mar 2016.

Alexander, M. (2012). *New Jim Crow: Mass incarceration in the age of colorblindness*. New York: The New Press.

Alkire, S. (2001). *Valuing freedoms: Sen's capability approach and poverty reduction*. Oxford: Oxford University Press.

H. Seckinelgin, *The Politics of Global AIDS*, Social Aspects of HIV 3,
DOI 10.1007/978-3-319-46013-0

Altman, D. (1971/1993). *Homosexual oppression and liberation*. London: Serpent's Tail.

Altman, D. (1994). *Power and community: Organizational and cultural responses to AIDS*. London: Taylor and Francis.

Altman, D., Aggleton, P., Williams, M., Kong, T., Reddy, V., Harrand, D., Reis, T., & Parker, R. (2012). Men who have sex with men: Stigma and discrimination. *Lancet*, 380(9839): 91–97.

AMSHER. (2016). *Who we are*? http://amsher.org/who-we-are/about-amsher/. Accessed 10 Mar 2016.

Angrist, J. D., & Pischke, J.-S. (2010). The credibility revolution in empirical economics: How better research design is taking the co out of econometrics. *The Journal of Economic Perspectives, 24*(2), 3–30.

Anscombe, E. (2000/1957). *Intention* (2nd ed.). Cambridge, MA: Harvard University Press.

Auerbach, J. (2009). Transforming social structures and environments to help in HIV prevention. *Health Affairs, 28*(6), 1655–1665.

Auerbach, J. D., & Hoppe, T. A. (2015). Beyond "getting drugs into bodies": Social science perspectives on pre-exposure prophylaxis for HIV. *Journal of the International AIDS Society, 18*(Suppl. 3), 19983.

Auerbach, J., Parkhurst, J. O., & Cáceres, C. F. (2011). Addressing social drivers of HIV/AIDS for the long-term response: Conceptual and methodological considerations. *Global Public Health: An International Journal for Research, Policy and Practice, 6*(Suppl. 3), S293–S309.

Auvert, B.,Taljaard, D., Lagarde, E., Sobngwi- Tambekou, J., Sitta, R., & Puren, A. (2005). Randomized controlled intervention trial of male circumcision for reduction of HIV risk: The ANRS 1265 trial. Plos/Medicine. http://journals.plos.org/plosmedicine/article?id=10.1371/journal.pmed.0020298. Accessed 2 Apr 2016.

Bailey, R. C., Moses, S., Parker, C. B., Agot, K., Maclean, I., Krieger, J. N., Williams, C. F., Campbell, R. T., & Ndinya-Achola, J. O. (2007). Male circumcision for HIB prevention in your men in Kisumu, Kenya: A randomised controlled trial. *Lancet, 369*(9562), 643–56.

Baldwin, P. (2005). *Disease and democracy: The industrialized world faces AIDS*. Berkeley: University of California Press.

Banarjee, A., & Duflo, E. (2010). Giving credit where it is due. *The Journal of Economic Perspectives, 24*(3), 61–79.

Baral, S. D. (2011). A cross-sectional assessment of the burden of HIV and associated individual- and structural-level characteristics among men who have sex with men in Swaziland. *Journal of International Aids Society, 16*(4 Suppl. 3), 18768.

Barker, G. (2003). *How do we know if men have changed? Promoting and measuring attitude change with young men*. Lessons from Programme H in Latin America [online]. Available from: http://www.un.org/womenwatch/daw/egm/men-boys2003/OP2-Barker.pdf. Accessed 15 Feb 2016.

Barre-Sinoussi, F., Chermann, J. C., Rey, F., et al. (1983). Isolation of a T-lymphotropic retrovirus from a patient at risk for acquired immune deficiency syndrome (AIDS). *Science, 220*, 868–71.

Barrett, S. M. (2004). Implementation studies: Time for a revival? Personal reflections on 20 years of implementation studies. *Public Administration, 82*(2), 249–262.

Barrett, C. B., & Carter, M. R. (2010). The power and pitfalls of experiments in development economics: Some non-random reflections. *Applied Economic Perspectives and Policy, 32*, 515–548.

BBC. (2009). *Scrap tests 'to boost HIV care'* 9 December 2009. http://news.bbc.co.uk/1/hi/health/8401681.stm. Accessed 10 Jan 2010.

Berkman, A., Garcia, G., Muñoz-Laboy, M., Paiva, V., & Parker, R. (2005). A critical analysis of the Brazilian response to HIV/AIDS: Lessons learned for controlling and mitigating the epidemic in developing countries. *American Journal of Public Health, 95*(7), 1162–1172.

Biehl, J. (2009). *Will to live: AIDS therapies and the politics of survival*. Princeton: Princeton University Press.

Blankenship, K. M., Bray, S. J., & Merson, M. H. (2000). Structural interventions in public health. *AIDS, 14*(Suppl. 1), S11–S21.

Bonnel, R., Rodriguez-Garcia, R., & Olivier, J. (2013). *Funding mechanisms for civil society: The experience of the AIDS response*. Washington, DC: World Bank.

Bosso, C. J. (1994). The contextual bases of problem definition. In D. A. Rochefort & R. W. Cobb (Eds.), *The politics of problem definition: Shaping the political agenda* (pp. 182–203). Lawrence: Kansas University Press.

Bourdieu, P. (1990). *The logic of practice*. Stanford: Stanford University Press.

Boyce, P. (2012). The ambivalent sexual subject: HIV prevention and male-to-male intimacy. In P. Aggleton, P. Boyce, H. L. Moore, & R. Parker (Eds.), *Understanding global sexualities: New frontiers* (pp. 75–88). London: Routledge.

Boyle, G. J., & Hill, G. (2011). Sub-Saharan African randomised clinical trials into male circumcision and HIV transmission: Methodological, ethical and legal concerns. *Journal of Law and Medicine, 19*(2), 316–34.

Broome, A., & Seabrooke, L. (2015). Shaping policy curves: Cognitive authority in transnational capacity building. *Public Administration, 93*(4), 956–972.

Brown, M. P. (1997). *RePlacing citizenship: AIDS activism and radial democracy*. London: Guilford Press.

Brown, W. (2015). *Undoing the demos: Neoliberalism's stealth revolution*. New York: Zone Books.

Buchbinder, S. P., & Liu, A. Y. (2015). CROI 2015: Advances in HIV testing and prevention strategies. *Topics in Antiviral Medicine, 23*(1), 8–27.

Buse, K., Dickinson, C., & Sidibé, M. (2008). HIV: Know your epidemic, act on its politics. *Journal of the Royal Society of Medicine, 101*, 572–573.

Cáceres, C. F., Koechlin, F., Goicochea, P., Sow, P., O'Reilly, K. R., Mayer, K. H., & Godfrey-Faussett, P. (2015). The promises and challenges of pre-exposure prophylaxis as part of the emerging paradigm of combination HIV prevention. *Journal of the International AIDS Society, 18*(Suppl. 3), 19949.

Callon, M., Lascoumes, P., & Barthe, Y. (2009). *Acting in an uncertain world: An essay on technical democracy*. Cambridge, MA: The MIT Press.

Campbell, C. (2013). Building 'HIV competent communities' in resource poor settings: Creating contexts that enable effective community mobilization. In R. A. Smith (Ed.), *Global HIV/AIDS politics, policy and activism: Persistent challenges and emerging issues* (pp. 107–134). New York: Praeger.

Canguilhem, G. (2012). *Writings on medicine* (S. Geroulanos & T. Meters, Trans.). New York: Fordham University Press.

Caron, D. (2014). *The nearness of others: Searching for tact and contact in the age of HIV*. London: University of Minnesota Press.

Cartwright, N. D. (2010). Will this policy work for you? Predicting effectiveness better: How philosophy helps. *Speech presented at PSA Presidential Address, Montreal, Canada, November 2010*.

Cartwright, N. (2011). The art medicine: A philosopher's view of the long road from RCTs to effectiveness. *Lancet, 377*, 1400–1401.

Cartwright, N., & Hardie, J. (2012). *Evidence-based policy: A critical guide to doing it better*. New York: Oxford University Press.

Castells, M. (2009). *The communication power*. New York: Oxford University Press.

Chandler, C. L. (2011). Creating a different international HIV response for young people. *Global Public Health: An International Journal for Research, Policy and Practice, 6*(Suppl. 3), S344–S356.

Chekel, J. (2005). International institutions and socialization in Europe: Introduction and framework. *International Organizations, 59*(4), 801–826.

Clarke, A. E., Shim, J. K., Mamo, L., Fosket, J. R., & Fishman, J. R. (2010). Biomedicalization. In A. E. Clarke, L. Mamo, J. R. Fosket, J. R. Fishman, & J. K. Shim (Eds.), *Biomedicalization: Technoscience, health and illness in the U.S*. London: Duke University Press.

Cobb, J. (2016, March 14). The matter of black lives: A new kind of movement found its moment. What will its future be? *The New Yorker*, pp. 34–40.

Cohen, J. (1997). The rise and fall of project SIDA. *Science, 278*(5343), 1565–1568.

Cohen, P. F. (1998). *Love and anger: Essay on AIDS activism and politics*. New York: Routledge.

Cohen, J., & Easterly, W. (2009). Introduction: Thinking big versus thinking small. In J. Cohen & W. Easterly (Eds.), *What works in development? Thinking big and thinking small*. Washington, DC: The Brookings Institution.

Connell, R. W. (1995). *Masculinities*. London: Polity.

Corrêa, S., Petchesky, R., & Parker, R. (2008). *Sexuality, health and human rights*. London: Routledge.

Coutinho, A., Roxo, U., Epino, H., Muganzi, A., Dorward, E., & Pick, B. (2012). The expanding role of civil society in the global HIV/AIDS response: What has the President's Emergency Program For AIDS Relief's role been? *AIDS, 60*(Suppl 3), S152–S157.

Crozier, M. P. (2010). Rethinking systems: Configurations of politics and policy in contemporary governance. *Administration and Society, 42*, 504–525.

Dart Trial Team. (2010). Routine versus clinically driven laboratory monitoring of HIV antiretroviral therapy in Africa (DART): A randomized non-inferiority trial. *Lancet, 375*, 123–131.

Deacon, A. (2010). Understanding the mechanisms of economic development. *The Journal of Economic Perspectives, 24*(3), 3–16.

de Camargo, K. R., Jr., de Oliveira Mendonça, A. L., Perrey, C., & Giami, A. (2013). Male circumcision and HIV: A controversy study on facts and values. *Global Public Health, 8*, 769–783.

De la Dehesa, R., & Mukherjea, A. (2012). Building capacities and producing citizens: The biopolitics of HIV prevention in Brazil. *Contemporary Politics, 18*(2), 186–199.

Denver Principles. (1983). http://www.actupny.org/documents/Denver.html. Accessed 25 Mar 2015.

Descombes, V. (2014). *The institutions of meaning: A defense of anthropological holism*. Cambridge: Harvard University Press.

Dolowitz, D. P., & Marsh, D. (1996). Who learn what from whom? A review of the policy transfer literature. *Political Studies, 44*(2), 343–357.

Doyal, L., & Doyal, L. (2013). *Living with HIV and dying with AIDS: Diversity, inequlaity and human rights in the global pandemic*. London: Ashgate.

ECOSOC. (1994). *Joint and co-sponsored United Nations programme on human immunodeficiency virus/acquired immunodeficiency syndrome (HIV/AIDS)*. http://www.un.org/documents/ecosoc/res/1994/eres1994-24.htm. Accessed 15 Feb 2015.

ECOSOC. (1995). E/1995L.24/Rev.1. Accessed 15 Feb 2015.

Edwards, M. (2009). *Civil society* (2nd ed.). London: Polity Press.

Elbe, S. (2010). *Security and global health: Toward the medicalization of insecurity*. Cambridge: Polity Press.

Epprecht, M. (2008). *Heterosexual Africa? The history of an idea from the age of exploration to the age of AIDS*. Athens: Ohio University Press.

Epstein, S. (1996). *Impure science: AIDS, activism and the politics of knowledge*. Berkeley: University of California Press.

Epstein, S. (2007). *Inclusion: The politics of difference in medical research*. Chicago: University of Chicago Press.

Eribon, D. (2004). *Insult and the making of gay self* (Michael Lucey, Trans.). Durham: Duke University Press.

Evans, M., & Davies, J. (1999). Understanding policy transfer: A multi-level, multi-disciplinary perspective. *Public Administration, 77*(2), 361–85.

Farmer, P. (2006). *AIDS and accusation: Haiti and the geography of blame*. Berkeley: University of California Press.

Fassin, D., & Pandolfi, M. (2010). Introduction: Military and humanitarian government, in the age of intervention. In D. Fassin & M. Pandolfi (Eds.), *Contemporary states of emergency: The politics of military and humanitarian interventions* (pp. 9–28). New York: Zone Books.

Fem-Prep. (2016, April 15). *Fem-Prep*. http://www.aidsmap.com/The-FEM-PrEP-study/page/1821879/Fem-PreP

Finnemore, M., & Sikkink, K. (1998). International norm dynamics and political change. *International Organizations, 52*(4), 887–917.

Flikschuh, K. (2014). The idea of philosophical fieldwork: Global justice, moral ignorance, intellectual attitudes. *Journal of Political Philosophy, 22*(1), 1–26.

Fogarty International Centre of US National Institutes of Health. (2016, April 26). *Implementation Science*. https://www.fic.nih.gov/researchtopics/pages/implementationscience.aspx

Foley, E. E., & Hendrixson, A. (2011). From population control to AIDS: Conceptualising and critique the global crisis model. *Global Public Health: An International Journal for Research, Policy and Practice, 6*(Suppl. 3), S310–S322.

Fox, A. M., Goldberg, A. B., Gore, R. J., & Bäringhausen, T. (2011). Conceptual and methodological challenges to measuring political commitment to respond to HIV. *Journal of the International AIDS Society, 14*(Suppl. 2), S2–S5.

Freyburg, T. (2015). Transgovernmental networks as an apprenticeship in democracy? Socialization into democratic governance through cross-national actvities. *International Studies Quarterly, 59*, 59–72.

Fried, L. P., Piot, P., Spencer, H. C., & Parker, R. (2012). The changing landscape of global public health. *Global Public Health, 7*(Suppl 1), S1–S4.

Gaudio, R. P. (2009). *Allah made us: Sexual outlaws in an Islamic African city*. Hoboken: Wiley-Blackwell.

Geertz, C. (1973). *The interpretation of cultures*. New York: Basic Books.

Gellner, E. (1994). *Conditions of liberty: Civil society and its rivals*. London: Allen Lane.

Geroulanos, S., & Meters, T. (2012). Introduction: George Canguilhem's critique of medical reason. In G. Canguilhem (Ed.), *Writings on medicine* (S. Geroulanos & T. Meters, Trans.). New York: Fordham University Press.

Giddens, A. (1984). *The constitution of society: Outline of the theory of structuration*. Cambridge: Polity Press.

Goffman, E. (1961). *The presentation of self in everyday life*. London: Penguin.

Goffman, E. (1968). *Stigma*. London: Penguin.

Gomez, J. E. (2015). Understanding the BRIC response to AIDS: Political institutions, civil society, and historical policy backlash in comparative perspective. *Commonwealth and Comparative Politics, 53*(3), 315–340.

Gordenker, L., Coate, R. A., Jönsson, C., & Söderholm, P. (1995). *International cooperation in response to AIDS*. London: Pinter.

Gorna, R. (2014). The architecture of AIDS. In *AIDS Today: Tell no lies and claim no easy victories* (pp. 97–114) 2014 Edition. Sussex: International HIV/AIDS Alliance.

Gould, D. B. (2009). *Moving politics: Emotion and ACT UP's fight against AIDS*. Chicago: University of Chicago Press.

Gray, R. H., Kigozi, G., Sewadda, D., Makumbi, F., Watya, S., Nalugoda, F., Kiwanuka, N., Moulton, L. H., Chaudhary, M. A., Chen, M. Z., Sewankambo, N. K., Wabwire-Mangen, F., Bacon, M. C., Williams, C. F. M., Opendi, P., Reynolds, S. J., Laeyendecker, O., Quinn, T. C., & Wawer, M. J. (2007). Male circumcision for HIV prevention in men in Rakai, Uganda: A randomised trial. *Lancet, 369*(9562), 657–66.

Groopman, J. (2014, December 22). Can AIDS be cured? What the battle's next stage will look like. *The New Yorker*.

Gupta, R. G., Parkhurst, J. O., Ogden, J. A., Aggleton, P., & Mahal, A. (2008). Structural approaches to HIV prevention. *Lancet, 372*(9640), 764–75.

Gupta, R. G., Ogden, J., & Warner, A. (2011). Moving forward on women's gender-related HIV vulnerability: The good news, the bad, and what to do about it. *Global Public Health: An International Journal for Research, Policy and Practice, 6*(Suppl. 3), S370–S382.

Gusfield, J. (1981). *The culture of public problems: Drinking-driving and the symbolic order*. Chicago: University of Chicago Press.

Hacking, I. (1995). The looping effects of human kinds. In D. Sperber, D. Premarck, & A. Premack (Eds.), *Causal cognition: An interdisciplinary approach*. Oxford: Oxford University Press.

Halperin, D. (2014). *How to be gay*. Cambridge, MA: Belknap Press.

Hankins, C. A., & de Zalduondo, B. O. (2010). Combination prevention: A deeper understanding of effective HIV prevention. *AIDS, 24*, S70–80.

Hankins, C., Macklin, R., & Warren, M. (2015). Translating PrEP effectiveness into public health impact: Key considerations for decision-makers on cost-effectiveness, price, regulatory issues, distributive justice and advocacy for access. *Journal of the International AIDS Society, 18*(Suppl. 3), 19973.

Harman, S. (2010). *The World Bank and HIV/AIDS: Setting a global agenda*. London: Routledge.

Harrison, G. W. (2011). Randomisation and its discontents. *Journal of African Economies, 20*, 626–652.

Hart, K. (2015). *Economy for and against democracy*. New York: Berghahn Books.

Harvard Consensus Statement. (2001). http://www.cid.harvard.edu/cidinthenews/pr/consensus_aids_therapy.pdf. Accessed 15 Feb 2015.

Heywood, M. (2014). Unravelling the human rights response. In *AIDS today: Tell no lies and claim no easy victories* (2014th ed., pp. 9–22). Sussex: International HIV/AIDS Alliance.

Higgins, J. A., Hoffman, S., & Dworkin, S. L. (2010). Rethinking gender, heterosexual men, and women's vulnerability to HIV/AIDS. *American Journal of Public Health, 100*(3), 435–445.

Hildebrandt, T. (2011). The political economy of social organization registration in China. *China Quarterly, 208*, 970–989.

Hisschemöller, M., Hoppe, R., Groenewegen, P., & Midden, C. (2001). Knowledge use and political choice in Dutch environmental policy: A problem structuring perspective on real life experiments in extended peer review. In M. Hisshemöller, R. Hoppe, W. N. Dunn, & J. Reavetz (Eds.), *Knowledge power and participation in environmental policy analysis* (pp. 47–72). New Brunswick: Transaction Publishers.

Holston, J. (2009). Insurgent citizenship in an era of global urban peripheries. *City and Society, 21*(2), 245–267.

Hoppe, R. (2011). *The governance of problems: Puzzling, powering and participation*. Bristol: The Policy Press.

Huysmans, J. (1995). Migrants as a security problem: Dangers of 'securitizing' societal issues. In R. Miles & D. Thranhardt (Eds.), *Migration and European integration: Dynamics of inclusion and exclusion* (pp. 53–72). London: Pinter.

ILGA. (2011). *The homophobic disruption of AMSHER's Pre-ICASA meeting – What really happened*. http://ilga.org/the-homphobic-disruption-of-amsher-s-pre-icasa-meeting-what-really--happened/. Accessed 15 Feb 2016.

Jain, S. L. (2010). The mortality effect: Counting the dead in the cancer trials. *Public Culture, 22*(1), 89–117.

Kallings, L., & McClure, C. (2008). *20 years of the international AIDS society: HIV professionals working together to fight AIDS*. Geneva: IAS. https://www.iasociety.org/Web/WebContent/File/IAS_20yearsIAS_book.pdf. Accessed 20 Dec 2015.

Keane, M. P. (2010). A structural perspective on the experimentalist school. *The Journal of Economic Perspectives, 24*(2), 47–58.

Kebaabetswe, P. M., Stirratt, M. J., McLellan-Lemal, E., Gray, S. C., Rose, C. E., Williams, T., et al. (2015). Factors Associated with Adherence and Conordance Between Measurtement Strategies in an HIV Daily Oral Tenofovir/Emtricitibine as Pre-exposure Prophylaxis (Prep) Clinical Trial, Botswana, 2007–2010. *AIDS and Behaviour, 19*(5), 758–769.

Keck, M. E., & Sikkink, K. (1998). *Activists beyond borders: Advocacy networks in international politics*. Ithaca: Cornell University Press.

Kim, J. Y., & Ammann, A. (2004). Is the "3by 5" initiative the best approach to tackling the HIV pandemic? *The Plos Debate*. http://journals.plos.org/plosmedicine/article?id=10.1371/journal.pmed.0010037. Accessed 15 Mar 2014.

Kingdon, J. (1995). *Agendas, alternatives and public policies* (2nd ed.). New York: Longman.

Kippax, S., & Holt, M. (2009). *The state of social and political science research related to HIV: A report for the international AIDS society*. Geneva: IAS.

Knutsson, B. (2016). Responsible risk taking: The neoliberal biopolitics of people living with HIV/AIDS in Rwanda. *Development and change* (Article first published online, pp. 1–25). Accessed 28 Mar 2016.

Kosseleck, R. (2002). *The practice of conceptual history: Timing history, spacing concepts* (T. Samuel Presner and others, Trans.). Stanford: Stanford University Press.

Kruse, J., & Martens, K. (2015). NGOs as actors in global social governance. In A. Kaasch & K. Martens (Eds.), *Actors and agency in global social governance*. Oxford: Oxford University Press.

Lambert, H. (2009). Evidentiary truths? The evidence of anthropology through the anthropology of medical evidence. *Anthropology Today, 25*(1), 16–20.

Larson, H. J., Bertozzi, S., & Piot, P. (2011). Redesigning the AIDS for long-term impact bulletin of the world health organization. http://www.who.int/bulletin/volumes/89/11/11-087114/en/. Accessed 20 Oct 2014.

Latour, B. (1987). *Science in action*. Cambridge, MA: Harvard University Press.

Lewis, D. (2014). *Non-governmental organizations, management and development*. Abington: Routledge.

Lisk, F. (2010). *Global institutions and the HIV/AIDS epidemic: Responding to an international crisis*. London: Routledge.

List, J. A. (2011). Why economists should conduct field experiments and 14 tips for pulling one off. *The Journal of Economic Perspectives, 25*(3), 3–16.

Lock, M., & Nguyen, V.-K. (2010). *An anthropology of medicine*. London: Wiley-Blackwell.

Long, N. (1992). Introduction. In N. Long & A. Long (Eds.), *Battlefields of knowledge: The interlocking of theory and practice in social research and development* (pp. 3–15). London: Routledge.

Longino, H. E. (2013). *Studying human behavior: How scientists investigate aggression & sexuality*. Chicago: The University of Chicago Press.

Ludwig, J., Kling, J. R., & Mullainathan, S. (2011). Mechanism experiments and policy evaluations'. *The Journal of Economic Perspectives, 25*(3), 17–38.

Luhmann, N. (1998). *Observations on modernity* (W. Whobrey, Trans.). Stanford: Stanford University Press.

Maartens, G., Celum, C., & Lewin, S. R. (2014). HIV infection: Epidemiology, pathogenesis, treatment, and prevention. *Lancet, 384*, 258–271.

Mambaonline. (2011). *MSM & HIV Pre- conference set for Ethiopia*. http://www.mambaonline.com/article.asp?artid=6357. Accessed 15 Feb 2016.

Mbali, M. (2013). *South African AIDS activism and global health politics*. London: Palgrave.

McCabe, L. (2007). Translating policy and practice day care for people with dementia in Kerala, India. *Global Social Policy, 7*(2), 203–221.

McFalls, L. (2010). Benevolent dictatorship: The formal logic of humanitarian government. In D. Fassin & M. Pandolfi (Eds.), *Contemporary states of emergency: The politics of military and humanitarian interventions* (pp. 317–334). New York: Zone Books.

McGoey, L. (2015). *No such thing as a free gift: The gates foundation and the price of philanthropy*. London: Verso.

MMWR. (1981). June 5. *Pneumocystis* Pneumonia – Los Angeles, *30*(21), 1–3.

MMWR. (1982). November 05, 31(43) 577–580 current trends acquired immune deficiency syndrome (AIDS): Precautions for clinical and laboratory staffs.

MMWR. (1983). March 04, 1983 32(8) current trends prevention of acquired immune deficiency syndrome (AIDS): Report of inter-agency recommendations.

Molina, J.-M., Capitant, C., Spire, B., Pialoux, G., Cotte, L., Charreau, I., Tremblay, C., Le Gall, J.-M., Cua, E., Pasquet, A., Raffi, F., Pintado, C., Chidiac, C., Chas, J., Charbonneau, P., Delaugerre, C., Suzan-Monti, M., Loze, B., Fonsart, J., Peytavin, G., Cheret, A., Timsit, J., Girard, G., Lorente, N., Préau, M., Rooney, J. F., Wainberg, M. A., Thompson, D., Rozenbaum, W., Doré, V., Marchand, L., Simon, M.-C., Etien, N., Aboulker, J.-P., Meyer, L., & Delfraissy,

J.-F. for the ANRS IPERGAY Study Group. (2015). On-demand preexposure prophylaxis in men at high risk for HIV-1 infection. *New England Journal of Medicine, 373*(23), 2237–2246.

Morell, R. (Ed.). (2001). *Changing men in Southern Africa*. London: Zed Books.

Mosse, D., & Lewis, D. (2006). Theoretical approaches to brokerage and translation in development. In D. Lewis & D. Mosse (Eds.), *Development brokers and translators: The ethnography of aid and agencies* (pp. 1–26). Bloomfield: Kumarian Press.

MoU. (1995). *Memorandum of understanding on a joint and cosponsored United Nations programme on HIV/AIDS*. http://www.ilo.org/public/english/bureau/leg/agreements/unaids.htm . Accessed 20 Mar 2015.

MRC. (2009). 'Thousands more could be treated for HIV in Africa if expensive routine lab tests are dropped' Medical Research Council Press Release MRC59/09. http://www.ctu.mrc.ac.uk/news_and_press_releases/news_archive/dart_trial_results_p… Accessed 15 Jan 2010.

Msimang, S. (2014). Executive summary. In *AIDS Today: Tell no lies and claim no easy victories 2014 edition* (pp. 3–7). Sussex: International HIV/AIDS Alliance.

MSMGF. (2016a). *MSMGF turns 10 in 2016*. http://msmgf.org/msmgf-turns-10-in-2016-save-the-date-and-help-us-celebrate/#ixzz40Exlv3zM. Accessed 21 Mar 2016.

MSMGF. (2016b). *Who are we*? http://msmgf.org/about-us/who-we-are/#ixzz40EwAiYAo . Accessed 21 Mar 2016.

Nair, S. (2013). Governance, representation and international aid. *Third World Quarterly, 34*(4), 630–652.

Nguyen, V.-K. (2010). *The republic of therapy: Triage and sovereignty in West Africa's of AIDS*. Durham: Duke University Press.

Ogden, J., Gupta, R. G., Fisher, W. F., & Warner, A. (2011a). Looking back, moving forward: Towards a game-changing response to AIDS. *Global Public Health: An International Journal for Research, Policy and Practice, 6*(Suppl. 3), S285–S292.

Ogden, J., Gupta, R. G., Warner, A., & Fisher, W. F. (2011b). Revolutionising the AIDS response. *Global Public Health: An International Journal for Research, Policy and Practice, 6*(Suppl. 3), S383–S395.

Ophir, A. (2010). The politics of catastrophization: Emergency and exception. In D. Fassin & M. Pandolfi (Eds.), *Contemporary states of emergency: The politics of military and humanitarian interventions* (pp. 59–88). New York: Zone Books.

O'Toole, L. J., Jr. (2004). The theory-practice issue in policy implementation research. *Public Administration, 82*(2), 309–329.

Pape, U. (2014). *The politics of HIV/AIDS in Russia*. London: Routledge.

Parker, R. (2002). The global HIV/AIDS pandemic, structural inequalities and the politics if international health. *American Journal of Public Health, 92*(3), 343–347.

Parker, R. (2009). Civil society, political mobilization, and the impact of HIV scale-up on health systems in Brazil. *Journal of Acquired Immune Deficiency Syndrome, 52*(Suppl. 1), S49–S51.

Parker, G. R., Easton, D., & Klein, C. H. (2000). Structural barriers and facilitators in HIV prevention: A review of international research. *AIDS, 14*(Suppl. 1), S22–S32.

Parkhurst, J. (2014). Structural approaches for prevention of sexually transmitted HIV in general populations: Definitions and an operational approach. *Journal of International AIDS Society, 17*, 19052.

Parkhurst, J. O., Chilongozi, D., & Hutchinson, E. (2015). Doubt, defiance, and identity: Understanding resistance to male circumcision for HIV prevention in Malawi. *Social Science & Medicine, 135*, 15–22.

Patten, S., Mantell, J., & Stein, Z. (2013). Discord and harmony in biomedical HIV prevention technologies: Advancements through advocacy. In R. A. Smith (Rd.), *Global HIV/AIDS politics, policy and activism: Persistent challenges and emerging issues* (pp. 73–106). New York: Praeger.

Patton, C. (1990). *Inventing AIDS*. London: Routledge.

Patton, C. (1996). *Fatal advise: How safe-sex education went wrong*. Durham: Duke University Press.

Paxton, N. A. (2012). Political science(s) and HIV: A critical analysis. *Contemporary Politics, 18*(2), 141–155.

PEPFAR. (2012, March 12). *PEPFAR's best practice's for volunatry medical male circumcision site operations*. https://www.usaid.gov/sites/default/files/documents/1864/pepfar_best_practice_for_vmmc_site_operations.pdf

Pereira, R. J. R. (2013). Sustainability in the post-PEPFAR period: Examples from Botswana, Ethiopia and South Africa. In R. A. Smith (Ed.), *Global HIV/AIDS politics, policy and activism: Persistent challenges and emerging issues* (pp. 27–44). New York: Praeger.

Petryna, A. (2009). *When experiments travel: Clinical trials and the global search for human subjects*. Princeton: Princeton University Press.

Piot, P. (2001). An interview with an interview with Dr. Peter Piot, Executive Director of UNAIDS Peter Piot and Shoma Chatterjee. *Journal of International Affairs, 55*(1), 193–207.

Piot, P. (2003). *The 3 by 5 initiative*. http://www.who.int/3by5/about/en/. Accessed 15 Apr 2015.

Piot, P. (2006). AIDS: From crisis management to sustained strategic response. *Lancet, 368*(9534), 526–30.

Piot, P. (2010). Setting new standards for targeted HIV prevention: The Avahan initiative in India. *Sex Transmitted Infections, 86*(1).

Piot, P., Quinn, T. C., Taelman, H., Feinsord, F. M., Minlangu, K. B., Wobin, O., Mbendi, N., Mazebo, P., Ndangi, K., Stevens, W., et al. (1984). Acquired immunodeficiency syndrome in a heterosexual population in Zaire. *Lancet, 2*(8394), 65–69.

Pisani, E. (2008). *The wisdom of whores: Bureaucrats, brothels and the business of AIDS*. London: Granta Books.

Power, J. (2015). *Movement, knowledge, emotion: Gay activism and HIV/AIDS in Australia*. Action: ANU Press.

Qureshi, A. (2015). AIDS activism in Pakistan: Diminishing funds, evasive state. *Development and Change, 64*(2), 320–338.

Race, K. (2003). Revaluation of risk among gay men. *AIDS Education and Prevention, 4*, 369–81.

Rancière, J. (2010). *Dissensus on politics and aesthetics*. London: Continuum.

Rao, P. J. V. R. (2010). Avahan: The transition to a publicly funded programme as a next stage. *Sexually Transmitted Infections, 86*(Suppl. 1), i7–i8.

Ravallion, M. (2009). Comment. In J. Cohen & W. Easterly (Eds.), *What works in development? Thinking big and thinking small* (pp. 51–54). Washington, DC: The Brookings Instituion.

Redfield, P. (2010). The verge of crisis: Doctors without borders in Uganda. In D. Fassin & M. Pandolfi (Eds.), *Contemporary states of emergency: The politics of military and humanitarian interventions* (pp. 173–196). New York: Zone Books.

Richey, L. A. (2008). *Population politics and development: From the policies to the clinics*. New York: Palgrave MacMillan.

Rodrik, D. (2009). The new development economics: We shall experiment, but how shall we learn? In J. Cohen & W. Easterly (Eds.), *What works in development?: Thinking big and thinking small*. Washington, DC: The Brookings Institution.

Rohleder, P., & Swartz, L. (2012). Disability, sexuality and sexual health. In P. Aggleton, P. Boyce, H. L. Moore, & R. Parker (Eds.), *Understanding global sexualities: New frontiers* (pp. 138–152). London: Routledge.

Rol, M., & Cartwright, N. (2012). Warranting the use of causal claims: A non-trivial case for interdisciplinarity. *Theoria, 74*, 189–202.

Rosengarten, M. (2009). *HIV interventions: Biomedicine and the traffic between information and flesh*. London: University of Washington Press.

Rothstein, B. (2009). Creating political legitimacy: Electoral democracy versus quality of government. *American Behavioral Scientist, 53*(3), 311–330.

Safaaids Meaningful Participation of People with AIDS (MIPA). http://www.safaids.net/files/MIPA_Brochure.pdf. Accessed 16 Feb 2016.

Scharpf, F. W. (1999). *Governing in Europe: Effective and democratic*. Oxford: Oxford University Press.

Schulman, S. (2013). *The gentrification of the mind: Witness to a lost imagination*. Berkeley: University of California Press.

Seabrooke, L. (2014). Epistemic arbitrage: Transnational professional knowledge in action. *Journal of Professions and Organization, 0*, 1–16.

Seckinelgin, H. (2002). Civil society as a metaphor for western liberalism. *Global Society, 16*(4), 357–376.

Seckinelgin, H. (2004). Between aspirations and assimilations: The world's poor meet the cosmopolitans. *Alternatives: Global, Local and Political, 29*(1), 69–88.

Seckinelgin, H. (2008). *International politics of HIV/AIDS: Global disease-local pain*. London: Routledge.

Seckinelgin, H. (2009a). Global social policy and international organizations linking social exclusion to durable inequality. *Global Social Policy, 9*(2), 205–227.

Seckinelgin, H. (2009b). Colonial silences, gender and sexuality: Unpacking international HIV and AIDS policy culture. In J. F. Klot & V.-K. Nguyen (Eds.), *The fourth wave: Violence, gender, culture and HIV in the 21st century*. Paris: UNESCO.

Seckinelgin, H. (2012a). *International security, conflict and gender 'HIV/AIDS is another war'*. London: Routledge.

Seckinelgin, H. (2012b). The global governance of success in HIV/AIDS policy: Emergency action, everyday lives and sen's capabilities. *Health and Place, 18*(3), 453–460.

Seeley, J., Watts, C. H., Kippax, S., Russell, S., Lori, H., & Whiteside, A. (2012). Addressing the structural drivers of HIV: A luxury or necessity for programmes? *AIDS, 15*(Suppl. 1), 17397.

Sen, A. (1992). *Inequality reexamined*. Oxford: Clarendon Press.

Sen, A. (2010). *The idea of justice*. London: Allen Lane.

Shadlen, K. C. (2013). Is AIDS treatment sustainable? In O. Aginam, J. Harrington, & P. K. Yu (Eds.), *The global governance of HIV/AIDS: Intellectual property and access to essential medicines* (pp. 29–58). Cheltenham: Edward Elgar.

Shaffer, P. (2011). Against excessive rhetoric in impact assessment: Overstating the case for randomised controlled experiments. *Journal of Development Studies, 47*, 1619–1635.

Shilts, R. (1988). *And the band played on: Politics, people, and the AIDS epidemic*. New York: St Martin.

Shriver, M. D., Everett, C., & Morin, F. S. (2000). Structural interventions to encourage primary HIV prevention among people living with HIV. *AIDS, 14*(Suppl. 1), S57–S62.

Sidibé, M., & Buse, K. (2009). Strength in unity. *Bulletin of the World Health Organization* 2009;87. http://www.who.int/bulletin/volumes/87/11/09-071621/en/. Accessed 15 Oct 2010.

Sidibé, M., & Buse, K. (2013a). AIDS governance: Best practices for a post-2015 world. *Lancet, 381*, 2147–49.

Sidibé, M., & Buse, K. (2013b). The response to the comments. *Lancet, 382*, 1018–1019.

Siplon, P. (2013). The troubled path to HIV/AIDS universal treatment access: Snatching defeat from the jaws of victory? In R. A. Smith (Ed.), *Global HIV/AIDS politics, policy and activism: Persistent challenges and emerging issues* (pp. 3–26). New York: Praeger.

Smith, R. A. (Ed.). (2013). *Global HIV/AIDS politics, policy and activism: Persistent challenges and emerging issues* (Vols. 1, 2, 3). Oxford: Praeger.

Smith, R. A., Parker, R. G., Garcia, J., & Remien, R. H. (2013). Social movement responses to HIV/AIDS in the United States and globality: Intersecting chronological, strategic, and health movement frames. In R. A. Smith (Ed.), *Global HIV/AIDS politics, policy and activism: Persistent challenges and emerging issues* (Vols. 1, 2, 3, pp. 3–44). Oxford: Praeger.

Strand, P. (2012). Public opinion as leadership disincentive: Exploring governance dilemma in eth AIDS response in Africa. *Contemporary Politics, 18*(2), 174–185.

Sumartojo, E. (2000). Structural factors in HIV prevention: Concepts, examples, and implications for research. *AIDS, 14*(Suppl. 1), S3–S10.

Taylor, C. (1971). Interpretation and the science of Man. In *Philosophy and the human sciences: Philosophical papers 2* (pp. 13–57). Cambridge: Cambridge University Press, 1985.

Taylor, S. W., Mayer, K. H., Elsesser, S. M., Mimiaga, M. J., O'Cleirigh, C., & Safren, S. A. (2014). Optimizing content for pre-exposure prophylaxis (PrEP) counseling for men who have sex with men: Perspectives of PrEP users and high-risk PrEP naïve men. *AIDS Behaviour, 18*(5), 871–879.

Teele, D. L. (Ed.). (2014). *Field experiments and their critics: Essays on the uses and abuses of experimentation in the social sciences*. New Haven: Yale University Press.
The Economist. (2014a). *Heal thyself*. December 2013. London.
The Economist. (2014b). *Too big to fail*. December 2013. London.
The Global Fund. (2016). Impact. http://www.theglobalfund.org/en/impact/. Accessed 5 Apr 2016.
The Lancet Commission. (2013). *Global health 2035*. http://globalhealth2035.org/report. Accessed 20 Feb 2016.
Thoreson, R. R. (2014). *Transnational LGBT activism: Working for sexual rights worldwide*. London: University of Minnesota Press.
Tillion, G. (2000). *Fragments de vie*. Paris: Éditions du Seuil.
Tilly, C. (2004). *Social movements, 1768–2004*. London: Routledge.
Tilly, C., & Tarrow, S. (2006). *Contentious politics*. Oxford: Oxford University Press.
Tocqueville, A. (2002). *Democracy in America* (2nd ed., H. C. Mansfield & D. Winthrop, Trans.). Chicago: University of Chicago Press.
Treichler, P. (1999). *How to have a theory in an epidemic: Cultural chronicles of AIDS*. Durham: Duke University Press.
UNAIDS. (1998). *The global HIV/AIDS epidemic- June 1998*. Geneva: UNAIDS.
UNAIDS. (1999a). *Financial and budgetary update Interim financial management information on 1998–1999*. UNAIDS/PCB (8)/99.3. http://www.unaids.org/sites/default/files/en/media/unaids/contentassets/dataimport/governance/pcb02/pcb_08_99_03_en.pdf. Accessed 28 Jan 2015.
UNAIDS. (1999b). *The AIDS report*. http://data.unaids.org/publications/irc-pub01/jc208-corpreport_en.pdf. Accessed 28 Jan 2015.
UNAIDS. (1999c). *From principle to practice: Greater involvement of people living with or affected by HIV/AIDS (GIPA)*. Best practice key material. http://data.unaids.org/pub/BriefingNote/2007/jc1299_policy_brief_gipa.pdf. Accessed 28 Jan 2015.
UNAIDS. (2001). *Declaration of commitment*. http://www.unaids.org/sites/default/files/sub_landing/files/aidsdeclaration_en.pdf. Accessed 28 Jan 2015.
UNAIDS. (2004). *Three ones*. Geneva: UNAIDS. http://www.unaids.org/en/about+unaids+/what+is+unaids/unaids+at+country+level/the+three+ones.asp. Accessed 28 Jan 2016.
UNAIDS. (2007). *Practical guidelines for intensifying HIV prevention: Towards universal access*. Geneva: UNAIDS.
UNAIDS. (2010). *UNAIDS report on the global AIDS epidemic 2010*. http://www.unaids.org/globalreport/Global_report.htm. Accessed 28 Jan 2015.
UNAIDS. (2012). *2012 UNAIDS report on the global epidemic*. Geneva: UNAIDS. http://www.unaids.org/en/resources/publications/2012/name,76121,en.asp. Accessed 28 Jan 2015.
UNAIDS. (2014). *90-90-90 An ambitious treatment target to help end the AIDS epidemic*. Geneva: UNAIDS.
UNAIDS. (2015a). *How AIDS changed everything*. Geneva: UNAIDS.
UNAIDS. (2015b). *Programme coordinating board-thirty seventh meeting*. http://www.unaids.org/sites/default/files/media_asset/20150930_UNAIDS_PCB37_Report-PCB36_EN.pdf. Accessed 28 Jan 2016.
UNAIDS. (2015c). *UNAIDS terminology guidelines 2015*. http://www.unaids.org/sites/default/files/media_asset/2015_terminology_guidelines_en.pdf. Accessed 28 Jan 2016.
UNAIDS. (2015d). *On the fast-track to end AIDS by 2030: Focus on location and population*. Geneva: UNAIDS.
UNAIDS. (2015e). *UNAIDS strategy 2016–2021*. Geneva: UNAIDS.
UNAIDS. (2016a). *2016 high-level on ending AIDS*. Geneva: UNAIDS.
UNAIDS. (2016b). *Invest in advocacy: Community participation in accountability is the key to ending the AIDS epidemic*. Geneva: UNAIDS.
UNAIDS and Lancet Commission. (2015). *Defeating AIDS, advancing global health*. London: *The lancet*. http://www.thelancet.com/journals/lancet/article/PIIS0140-6736%2815%. Accessed 5 Feb 2016.

Verhoeven, J. C. (1993). An interview with Erving Goffman 1980. *Research on Language & Social Interaction, 26*(3), 317–348.

Walker, J., & Ostrom, E. (2005). Trust and reciprocity as foundations of trust. In K. S. Cook, M. Levi, & R. Hardin (Eds.), *Whom can we trust?: How groups, networks, and institutions make trust possible*. New York: Russel Sage Foundation.

Walker, J., & Ostrom, E. (2009). Conclusion. In J. Walker & E. Ostrom (Eds.), *Trust and reciprocity interdisciplinary lessons for experimental research* (pp. 381–386). New York: Russel Sage Foundation.

Wamai, R. G., Morris, B. J., Waskett, J. H., Green, E. C., Banerjee, J., Bailey, R. C., Kalusner, J. D., Sokal, D. C., & Hankins, C. A. (2012). Critism of African trials fail to withsthand scrutiny: Male circumcision does prevent HIV infection. *Jounal of Law and Medicine, 20*(1), 93–123.

Wamai, R. G., Morris, B. J., Bailey, R. C., Kalusner, J. D., & Boedicker, M. N. (2015). Male circumcision for protection against HIV infection in sub-Saharn Africa: The evidence in favour justifies the implementation now in progress. *Global Public Health, 10*(5–6), 639–666.

Weiss, H. A., Dickson, K. E., Agot, K., & Hankins, C. A. (2010). Male circumcision for HIV prevention: Current research and programmatic issues. *AIDS, 24*(Suppl. 4), S61–S69.

WHO. (2003). *The 3 by 5 initiative*. http://www.who.int/3by5/about/initiative/en/. Accessed 15 Apr 2015.

WHO. (2007). WHO and UNAIDS announce recommendations from expert consultation on male circumcision for HIV prevention. *WHO*. http://www.who.int/hiv/mediacentre/news68/en/. Accessed 2 Apr 2016.

WHO. (2014). WHO progress report – Voluntary medical male circumcision for HIV prevention in priority countries of East and Southern Africa. *WHO*. http://www.who.int/hiv/topics/malecircumcision/male-circumcision-info-2014/en/. Accessed 2 Apr 2016.

WHO. (2015). *The guidelines on when to start antiretroviral therapy and on pre-exposure prophylaxis*. http://www.who.int/hiv/pub/guidelines/earlyrelease-arv/en/. Accessed 14 Mar 2016.

Whyte, S. R., Whyte, M. A., Meinert, L., & Twebaze, J. (2013). Therapeutic citizenship: Belonging in Uganda's projectified landscape of AIDS care. In J. Biehl & A. Petryna (Eds.), *When people come first: Critical studies in global health* (pp. 140–166). Oxford: Princeton University Press.

Wilson, D., & Halperin, D. T. (2008). Know your epidemic, know your response. *Lancet, 372*(9637), 423–426.

Wohlfeiler, D. (2000). Structural and environmental HIV prevention for gay and bisexual men. *AIDS, 14*(Suppl. 1), S52–S56.

Wolf, R. C., Cheng, A. S., Kapesa, L., & Castor, D. (2013). Building the evidence base for urgent action: HIV epidemiology and innovative programming for men who have sex with men in sub-Saharan Africa. *Journal of International AIDS Society, 16*(4 Supl 3), 18903.

Woods, N. (2006). *The globalizers: The IMF, the World Bank, and their barrowers*. Ithaca: Cornell University Press.

Woodling, M., Williams, O. D., & Rushton, S. (2012). New life in old frames: HIV, development and the 'AIDS plus MDGs' approach. *Global Health Public Health, 7*(Sup.2), S144–S155.

Woolcock, M. (2013). Using case studies to explore the external validity of 'complex' development interventions. *Evaluation, 19*(3), 229–248.

MIX
Papier aus verantwortungsvollen Quellen
Paper from responsible sources
FSC® C105338
FSC
www.fsc.org

If you have any concerns about our products,
you can contact us on
ProductSafety@springernature.com

In case Publisher is established outside the EU,
the EU authorized representative is:
Springer Nature Customer Service Center GmbH
Europaplatz 3, 69115 Heidelberg, Germany

Printed by Libri Plureos GmbH
in Hamburg, Germany